MW01479544

SUPERIOR BOOKS
#206 - 13308 - 76th Avenue
Surrey, B.C.   V3W 2W1
(604) 572-1065 Fax:(604) 572-1085

DR. ANNE'S JOURNAL

DR. ANNE'S JOURNAL

by Robert LLoyd Ph.D.

DAVAR PUBLISHING
P.O. Box 1100
Cannon Beach, OR 97110

First printing, May 1990

Library of Congress Catalog Card Number 90-81824
ISBN 0-937831-03-4

Manufactured in the United States of America

Cover model -- Alicia Harrison
Makeup artist -- Farah Darakhshi
Cover photo -- Don Little Photography
Cover design -- Berg Graphics

*My people
are destroyed
for lack of knowledge.
Hosea 4:6*

for Anne . . .

PROLOGUE

Washington, D.C. — A few minutes after midnight, the government limousine pulled to the entrance of Walter Reed Army Medical Center, where a nurse waited with her wheelchair patient. Moving with alacrity, the driver hastened to assist the patient. With a muttered thanks, the patient refused the man's hand and struggled to his feet unaided, while the nurse hovered uncertainly in the background.

Headlights from an arriving car momentarily illuminated the patient's visage, pale and drawn from suffering, highlighting a temple-to-jaw scar on the left side of the man's face.

Startled by the blinding light, he instinctively cupped his face with his hands, and for a single moment the beam magnified itself a thousand fold as it was reflected from the exquisite ring on the man's left hand. The size of the huge diamond was startling, but it was the setting that caught the eye: curiously-wrought by a master craftsman, the setting was a death's head, with the gem itself forming the skull.

Thrown off balance, the man took a single step, faltered and began to fall. *My God*, he thought, *the doctor was right . . . I am too weak to be out of bed.*

Instantly Fred was at his side, preventing the fall. Gently easing his charge into the limousine, he noted the sparse, greying stubble beginning to show on the man's head. Fred felt a pang of anger mixed with fear . . .

The man positioned himself with some difficulty, then half-spoke, half groaned, "Okay, Fred. Let's go!"

"Yes, sir . . ." Fred closed the door and slid behind the wheel. He drove fast, but carefully through the dark streets.

Scarcely aware of the ride, the doctor's words repeated themselves in his mind: *Colon cancer . . . latter stages . . . surgery . . . chemo. Radiation. Nothing more we can do. Just a matter of weeks, months at the most . . .*

Slumped painfully in the seat, he stared at the back of Fred's head, seeing nothing. *Too late? God, is it too late?*

An hour later the black limo paused briefly at the gate of an unnamed airport. Fred identified himself to the Marine guard, who waved him on. He gunned the vehicle to the awaiting Lear Jet. The vehicle barely stopped before the door popped open and the patient struggled out by himself.

Leaning heavily upon Fred, he hobbled painfully to the aircraft's boarding ladder. The cabin attendant reached down and took the man's hand.

Fred grabbed their luggage and boarded. One minute later the aircraft was in the air, its nose pointed southwest . . .

A private ambulance awaited them at San Diego. Though the patient was obviously tired, he refused the proffered wheelchair and, under Fred's watchful eye, doggedly moved to the ambulance under his own power.

Before the 405 Freeway became crowded with early morning commuters, the ambulance and its passengers had crossed the border into Mexico. Shortly thereafter, they arrived at a small, well-equipped clinic . . .

They were expected. Barely conscious by now, the patient was scarcely aware of the ministrations of the skilled professionals who undressed him and started his therapy.

Fred sought out the attending physician. His jaws white with the tension he felt, he asked, "Doc, do you think it's too late?"

The doctor's barely perceptible shrug spoke volumes.

Seeing that no better answer was forthcoming, Fred sighed. "He is to be registered as John Doe . . . all his expenses will be taken care of with cash . . ."

The doctor nodded and entered John Doe's room . . .

CHAPTER ONE

In the semi-darkness of his book-littered office,
the bluish glow of the monitor cast an eerie reflection
across the weary face of the man bent over his
computer; his full attention upon the content of the
white lines of words marching in orderly fashion and
precision across the glowing screen. The hour is late,
but to Benjamin Rush, time is completely relative,
and aside from planes to catch and deadlines to meet,
it has little meaning. He completes the page, scrolls
it back and reviews what he has written.

Satisfied at last, Ben prints out a draft copy of
the chapter, and with it in hand, makes his way to
the kitchen and brews himself a pot of tea to sip on
while he goes over it.

Frowning, he blue pencils several lines, deletes
some words and sentences, adds others. Then, intent
upon the sheaf of pages, cup in one hand, he heads
for the bedroom at the other wing of the house, to get
his wife's opinion. Suddenly, he pauses in mid stride,
a look of indescribable pain upon his face . . .

She's gone. Anne's not here anymore.

Afterwards, remembering this moment,
everything seemed to happen in slow motion. He
turns on his heel, strides back to the kitchen to
dispose of the tea, which he no longer wants. With a
groan wrung from deep within, he heedlessly drops
the papers on the table — and as though drawn by

an irresistible force, moves back to that room where she . . . where she . . . is, or *was*.

He pauses at the doorway, hesitant to enter. It is *her room*. Theirs, actually. But truly hers. Even now, after two years, the room is electric with her presence. Suffused with the light of her. Her warm smile. Her aura. It's like, like she has just stepped into another part of the house. And will be popping back at any moment . . .

For the first time since her death, he sleeps in that room that night . . .

Her scream awakens him. He sits up, disoriented. Then he sees her. She is running like a frightened rabbit across a vast clearing with the forest in the background. Her scream trembles on the wind. He leaps to his feet and runs after her. He *must* catch her, but he does not know why.

His feet pound across an open field. He runs, but she runs faster and stays ahead of him. Somehow he knows that she is trying to reach the safety of the grove of trees. She's wearing her loveliest nightgown: gossamer-thin, ethereal, and it billows out behind her as she runs, giving her the appearance of an angel. She is more beautiful than he'd remembered . . .

But she is terrified. Why is she so frightened?

He knows that he knows, but cannot force himself to remember. There it is: the shapeless, nameless *Thing*. That's why she is so frightened. It is between them, gaining on her. He has to reach her before the *Thing* catches her.

She is trying to run very fast, but it seems like her feet are moving in slow motion. And the *Thing*, the fearsome, hated *Thing* is running faster than both of them. It is gaining on her.

She *must* reach the other side before it catches her. He tries to call, to urge her to greater speed, but no words come. He tries to run faster, but his feet

suddenly are encased in concrete. They weigh tons.
He strains to move them, but can hardly lift them.

His heart pounds audibly.

She must have heard his heart pounding, for
she throws him a quick look over her shoulder. As
she does, she stumbles. She is panic-stricken and
cries out in fear. Her lips form the words, "Please
help me. Please!" But no words came out.

Oh, God, I've got to reach her. To help her.

"Anne . . . Dear Doctor Anne . . ." He is
awakened by the sound of his own voice.

He sits up. The room is empty. And the bed is
a jumble of sweaty, twisted bed coverings . . .
Comprehension comes. He beats his pillow with both
fists, sobbing.

The clock on the landing chimes: bong, bong,
bong. Three o'clock. He lies awake, remembering.

He must have dozed for the grey of dawn is
now filtering through his window. Ben staggers
wearily to the bathroom and turns on the shower full
force.

Another endless, lonely day had begun.

Hunched over his desk, blue pencil poised,
Ross Hannibal read rapidly and Ben marvelled at
how quickly the man could absorb in seconds the
sentences he had labored over for hours and days.
Neither man spoke while Hannibal scanned page
after page almost as fast as he could turn them. Ben
allowed his eyes to wander around the book-lined,
manuscript-filled working office of Cutting Edge
Publications' senior editor.

This was Ben's first time in Ross's office.
Though he was, like most writers, very alert
concerning the publishing scene, he had known little
about Cutting Edge before that telephone message
that had been left on his machine a month ago. "My
name is Ross Hannibal, Senior Editor of Cutting

Edge Publications. I'm familiar with your work. I'd like very much to discuss a book idea with you. Please call me."

Curious, Ben telephoned the next day.

To his amazement, Ross Hannibal answered the telephone himself. He came right to the point. "I've read your last couple of books. Like your style. How about lunch?"

"Where and when?"

"Do you like salads?"

"Sure."

"The Sea Lion in Malibu has a great salad bar. How about tomorrow? Eleven-thirty?"

"I know the place. Eleven thirty's fine."

"I like it here," Ross said the next day when they were seated at a window with a panoramic view of the Pacific from Palos Verdes Peninsula to Point Dume. "It rests my weary editor's eyes." He was wearing a short-sleeved shirt, open at the front, crumpled tan slacks and deck shoes.

They talked generally of books, editors and publishers until they finished their lunch. Then Ross said gently, "I understand you lost your wife recently . . ."

Ben looked up sharply. "How did you know?"

"Carolyn Kemp."

Ben puzzled with that momentarily. "Oh, the nurse. The one in Anne's office."

"Yes. She told me about Anne. She admired your wife greatly."

"So did I."

"I gathered that."

Ben stared at the breakers dashing spray upon their window, obviously not seeing them.

Ross cleared his throat. "Carolyn told me something else. That Anne kept a journal . . . sort of a medical diary . . ."

"Yes. She started it before we met. In med school."

8

"Have you read it?"

"Some . . ."

Ross studied Ben's somber face. "Have you considered doing any medical writing?"

"Yes . . . no. Well, not really. A few months after Anne's death . . . I still have difficulty with that word. Anyway, I picked it up from her desk. Read some . . ."

He drew a deep breath. ". . . But then, I put it down. I just wasn't ready . . ."

"And now?"

"I don't know. I just don't know."

Ross handed the waiter his credit card. "Carolyn told me that Anne had been doing a bit of independent research . . . about cancer. Said Anne recorded it all in her Journal . . ."

Ben nodded. "She recorded everything in her Journal. The patients she saw. Their diagnoses, prognoses . . . treatment modalities. Everything."

"Despite all that . . . it still got her. The cancer."

Ben nodded, unsmiling.

Ross signed the check and put his card away. He spoke the next words slowly, "Ben, please be candid with me. This may be an imposition, but . . . would you mind letting me look at your wife's Journal?"

Ben hesitated briefly. "What did you have in mind?"

"I'm not sure until I read it."

Ben ran his fingers through his thick curly hair. "Well, I don't think Anne would mind. I'll drop it in the mail."

That had been a week ago. Yesterday Ross had called. "Ben, I've just finished reading Anne's Journal. Like to talk to you about it. Would you stop by?"

"Sure. I'll be in the area this afternoon."

Cutting Edge Publishing, Inc., Ben had learned, had been formed by a consortium of angry consumers grown tired of the exponentially increasing abuses in the American health establishment, and had decided to fight back. They created Cutting Edge specifically to "expose medical and pharmaceutical malpractice, conspiracy and fraud wherever it exists." And in the process scouted around for a skilled, tough-minded editor who could handle the flak. The field soon narrowed to Ross Hannibal. He was willingly conscripted to head up Cutting Edge's editorial department.

An editor of the old school, Hannibal came up through the ranks. He earned his wings under fire in the South Pacific as a war correspondent, then returned to the University of Missouri and earned his doctorate from the School of Journalism, where he still taught a class in Investigative Journalism each summer. His students knew him to be tough and crusty, but fair; a man who obviously knew the business of writing and publishing from the inside out.

Hannibal was truly an editor's editor. In his spare time — "between the hours of two and four in the mornings," he said, half jokingly — he ground out at least one book a year; most made the *New York Times* Best Seller list. A vegetarian, Hannibal believed that half the world's ills were caused by what a man eats, and the other half by what he thinks. Widowed a dozen years ago, though in his mid-seventies, Hannibal kept in shape by swimming daily laps in his all-season pool and by bicycling at least fifty miles a week.

An avid sailor, Ben learned, Hannibal owned and frequently sailed his own 45-foot sloop, aptly named, "The Blue Pencil," that he kept docked in a Marina Del Rey slip.

Ross rose when Ben entered, still wearing the same crumpled tan slacks and deck shoes. He waved Ben to a chair. "What have you got there?"

"Thought you might like to glance at this," Ben said, handing Hannibal a large manila envelope. "Some thoughts that came when I was perusing Anne's Journal. Pulled them out this morning. You might be interested . . ."

"Thanks." Ross opened the envelope and began reading rapidly.

Before Anne died she had told him he would know what to do with her Journal, ". . . when I am gone . . ." Was *this* what she meant? To open up to the world her most private self?

He looked up, suddenly aware that Ross had finished reading. He was not smiling.

"You sound angry."

"I was. Still am. The whole thing's a travesty . . ."

"What do you mean?"

"I think you know. You've read her Journal. You've caught the essence of her medical philosophy . . ." Ben shifted his position, recrossed his legs. "I happen to agree with her. And I think the public's got a right to know."

"Absolutely. Would you like to tell them?"

Ben stared at Hannibal. "Yes . . . no. I mean, I'm a writer, but I'm not a medical writer . . ."

"But you call yourself an investigative journalist."

"Yes."

"You've written some powerful books. Your face is familiar to TV audiences. Why don't you tell the world about Anne . . . about the needless way she died?"

Ben was aware that his hands had balled into fists and that he was tensely perched on the edge of his chair. His throat was dry, his stomach burned.

Why not tell the world about Anne? He drew a deep breath and released it.

"Maybe . . . maybe I would."

"Some of Anne's Journal is pretty heavy stuff."

"Heavy, yes. But well documented."

Ross removed his feet from his desk. "Okay, let's think about that for a minute. Frankly, Cutting Edge is interested in doing a book on alternative treatments for cancer. We've had it in mind for some time. With your permission, I'd like to include Anne's research."

He paused to let his words sink in. Ben felt his pulse thumping in his temples.

"At the risk of opening a fresh wound, I've got to ask you a couple of hard questions. Okay?"

Ben nodded, his face frozen.

"First question: In your opinion, if Anne had chosen the alternative therapy route to treat her lymphoma, do you believe that choice would have saved her life?"

The question sliced through Ben's bluff exterior like a new scalpel. He was caught off guard: It was like surgery without anesthetic. Raw, bleeding. He closed his eyes. And the film rolled . . .

It was an extraordinarily painful experience. The pictures were as sharp and clear as the day they were taken. Wrenchingly thin now, her head bristly with new growth of hair, Anne's green eyes, now sunken in her skeletal face, followed his every movement when he brought the tray into the room.

He bowed. "Doctor Anne, I presume. Breakfast is served."

She smiled wanly, "How lovely, Ben. I thank you. And . . . oh, how I love you . . ." Unbidden, a tear slid down upon the pillow. He placed the tray over her knees and uncovered the bowl of fresh-sliced strawberries, her favorite. She reached for his hand, then patted the bed beside her.

"Please, Ben. Sit down."

He sat beside her on the bed. She toyed briefly with her spoon then put it down. "I'm sorry, Ben . . . I, I can't. I'm not hungry. Please forgive me. It *looks* good. Really it does."

He nodded and tried to smile. While everything inside of him twisted and turned in rebellion. Why Anne? Oh, God, why Anne?

"Ben, we must talk . . . I mean, I must talk. And you must listen . . ." She looked up into his face. "Okay?"

"Yes, my love . . . I know." He took a deep breath, held it, and released it slowly. "I am ready." He swallowed hard at the lie. He *was not* ready for what he believed was coming. And never would be ready. Never. Never . . .

"I must tell you about my Journal . . ."

She opened the thick, leather-bound book that showed signs of much use. "Ben, dear, dear, Ben," she began, "there is much in here that you need to know. And when . . ." She squeezed her eyes closed tightly.

"And when . . ." she went on, her voice stronger, ". . . when the time comes . . . then, you will know . . . you'll know what to do with it . . ."

"How will I know?" he asked, fighting the knot in his stomach that threatened to explode.

"You'll know, Ben. You'll just know. And then . . . then others can possibly be spared the . . . same . . . pain . . . that you and I . . ." Her resolve broke and she pulled Ben down to her, weeping convulsively. "Oh, Ben . . . I love you so . . ."

Ben attempted to notify Bertram Collins of his daughter's illness. A secretary informed him that "Mr. Collins is out of the country and is not expected back in his office for another few weeks . . . Shall I have him return the call?"

He hesitated. Not since Ben had known Anne had Collins initiated any kind of communication with his daughter.

"Sir . . ." the secretary's voice urged, "shall I have Mr. Collins return the call?"

"Uh, yes. Please tell him Ben Rush called to tell him that his daughter is very ill. She's in the hospital in Santa Monica . . . having surgery."

"I'll make sure he gets the message. Goodbye."

Sick at heart, Ben slowly replaced the instrument. He had little hope that Collins would return the call. But it had been important to Anne that he try to contact her father. After so many years of neglect, Ben wondered if Anne's life — or her death, for that matter — meant anything at all to Collins.

A week later, on a bright sunshiny day, the kind of day made for life, he stood beside her grave.

He opened his eyes. Hannibal smiled understandingly. "I'm sorry, Ben. Truly sorry. But, I had to ask . . ."

Ben was pale. His perspiration-drenched shirt clung to his body. Ross was aware that Ben was holding himself in tight rein. With hardly a pause, Ben answered.

"The answer, Ross . . . and it's like rubbing a raw nerve to tell you this, but the answer is yes. If Anne had chosen alternative modalities . . . I believe she'd be alive today."

Ross acknowledged his answer with a slight nod. "Now for the second question, Ben. In a way, it's even tougher than the first one."

Ross tapped Anne's Journal, "Then why, if you believe that, and if Anne believed it, why, in God's name didn't she go that route . . . and save her own life."

"Because," Ben forced the words through tight lips, "because of professional peer pressure, and . . ."

The unfinished sentence dangled between them.

"And . . .?" Hannibal probed gently.

Ben swallowed hard before forcing the words out. "And her father . . ."

"Her *father*?" Ross echoed in surprise. "Her father? Isn't her father an attorney? In San Francisco?"

"That's right. He was and is an attorney. The founder and senior partner of Collins, Gould and Adams. You know the firm?"

"Yes. But I don't understand. That shouldn't have made any difference . . . should it?" Hannibal's weather-beaten brow was furrowed.

"Shouldn't. But did. What you probably didn't know was that Collins' firm is retained by BII, Bullion, Inc., International, the largest manufacturer of cancer drugs in the world . . ."

"But, I still don't understand."

Tight-lipped, Ben said, "You would if you knew Bertram Collins . . ."

CHAPTER TWO

He had driven this back country road so often
that it required little conscious thought or effort,
which was good, because today he had little of either
available to expend. As he had told Ross Hannibal,
he *was* tired. Exhausted, really. It always took it out
of him to write a book, especially the one he'd just
completed. Two years of research and a full six
months at his computer had drained him. Actually,
he'd spent nearly three years of elapsed time in his
research, but he'd drastically curtailed his work when
Anne became critically ill.

For months after she died, he had done little
but mope around, too drained emotionally to write.
Finally and gradually his old drive returned and he
had picked up the loose ends and carried the
assignment to completion.

The road got rougher and he was forced to
give it more of his attention. He'd turned off the
coast highway thirty minutes ago and since then had
been climbing steadily, the gears of his old Land
Rover groaning in protest. Winding around the sharp
curves, he caught glimpses of the sun, partially
wrapped in pink-gold clouds, sinking into the Pacific.
Anne had loved this drive, and after long days caring
for her patients had looked forward to these moments
alone.

He loved the drive, too, but no longer looked forward to the solitude. That's all he had known these past two years . . .

Near the top of the hill, the driveway veered sharply to the right. Ben downshifted, and bounced around and through the chuck holes, cut by the late rains the county road-grader hadn't mended. Five minutes more and the cabin came into view. The last rays of the sun flashed gold from huge picture windows, and suddenly, as always, his heart bounded with anticipation. More even than their Santa Monica town house, this had been their home.

He urged the groaning vehicle around a final hill and through the grove of poplars, past the oleander windbreak, up to the two-car garage that housed her Mercedes that hadn't been driven for two years. He made a mental note to start it up and run it for a few minutes. Not tonight. Maybe tomorrow. Or the next day . . .

Tonight he would just . . . what would he do?

Suddenly unwilling to face the emptiness of the cabin, Ben shut off the engine and tiredly rested his head against the steering wheel. Dear God, why did she have to leave me?

He had found her, in of all places, a forest fire-fighting camp in Idaho. McCall, Idaho would have been the last place in the world he would ever have expected to spend a summer. Who had ever *heard* of McCall? It sounded like the name of a womens' magazine, not a prosperous Idaho summer lake resort. But there had been that note on the Pepperdine dorm bulletin board. "Fire fighters needed. Good pay." Except for an address and telephone number, that was all. He made application and promptly forgot.

A week later, surfeited with Malibu surfing, fed up with Pacific Coast Highway traffic, and unwilling to seek a summer job in downtown Los

Angeles, he came across the number again and promptly dialed it.

A pleasant, young-sounding female voice responded. "Yes," she said, "we got your application. You've been on my list to call this week. It's hot this summer. Hot and dry. Lots of fires. We need you. How soon can you come?"

"How about today?"

"Fine. I'll meet you at the bus."

"Bus? No airplane?"

"Mr. Rush, this place isn't exactly Los Angeles. You'll have to fly to Boise and take a Greyhound. It arrives twice a day. I meet both of them. Okay?"

"Sure. I'll be there as soon as I can catch a plane." He hesitated. "How will I know you?"

"I'll know you. Your picture. Remember?"

He'd never been to Idaho before and hadn't known what to expect. The tiny Boise airport intrigued him. And the Greyhound drive up the McCall River was delightful. The mountains and trees were different than anything he'd ever seen, and he was almost sorry when they finally wound their way through the hills and valleys and reached busy little McCall.

To the right, as they drove down the main street that was clogged with RVs, campers and out-of-state cars, was McCall Lake. A light breeze ruffled the surface into a million whitecaps. "It's beautiful," he said out loud.

"Can be dangerous," his seat mate volunteered. "Just don't let yourself get caught out there in a sudden squall. Waves get up to five, six feet within minutes. I know. Happened to me. Swamped me. Had to be rescued."

High above the far side of the lake on a mountaintop stood a spindly tower. "What's that?" he asked his knowledgeable friend.

"Fire lookout. Got them all around here on the high points."

19

Despite himself, a quiver of excitement ran through him. "Fire lookout? You mean somebody *lives* up there? All the time?"

"That's right. Twenty-four hours. It's been a dry summer. Fires get started from lightning. Careless campers. Smokers. Got to nip fires in the bud or they spread like . . . like wildfire. Well, I guess we're here. End of the line for me. You, too?"

"Yes." He began gathering up his gear.

"Vacation?"

"No. Fire fighting."

"Oh." The old man raised his eyebrows. "First time to fight fire?"

Ben grinned. "First time. Maybe the last."

"Well, keep alert. I've been on the fire line a hundred times. Hard work. Dirty work. I'm too old for that now. But I kinda liked it."

Ben stepped off the bus, squinting in the bright sunlight, and suddenly struck by the pervasive smell of wood smoke. A petite young woman, attractive in jeans and denim top smiled at him. "Mr. Rush. I'm Anne Collins."

"Oh, hi," he said in sudden confusion. "I expected someone older, I guess . . . more . . ."

"More mature?" Her eyes were steady, penetrating.

"I don't know. I guess I wasn't really thinking. But, I mean, are *you* a fire fighter? I thought only men . . ."

"Typical male attitude," she said, unsmiling. "I'm in pre-med at Stanford. Summer work in the Northwest appealed to me, so here I am. And, no, I don't fight fires. I'm the gal Friday. I answer the phones. Manage the office. Part-time dispatcher. All of that. And that's just part of my job description."

While she talked she was herding him toward the dusty-looking Bronco. "Toss your bags in the back. Jump in. I've got to get back to the office."

While she drove, expertly dodging the tourist traffic, he assessed her. He liked what he saw. She was pretty with her short, dark hair, stylishly cut close to her head. Petite. Sun-browned. With a smudge of soot on her cheek.

She turned and caught his eye. "Something wrong, Mister Rush?"

Despite himself the blood rushed to his face. "Please call me Ben. And, no, nothing's wrong. But, did you know you've got soot on your face. You must have been on the fire line."

She glanced in the mirror and dabbed at the spot. "Fallout from the fires," she explained. "They're all around us."

He nodded, remembering the wood smoke odor and the light haze that hung over the lake.

"Have you fought fires before, Ben?"

"First time."

"Do you know anything about fighting fires?"

"Nothing. I've just watched fire fighters on TV. That's all."

"It's hard work." She looked him over. "But you look fit enough."

"Thanks. I play tennis a lot. Surf. Work out four or five times a week. Try to stay in shape."

"Here we are. The office." She pointed. "Those are the bunk houses out back. I'll give you a key to your room. You'll be on the line at first light. Better catch a little sleep while you can."

Stretched out on his bunk an hour later, clad only in jockey shorts, he wiped the sweat from his face. Sleep, she'd said. But who could sleep in this heat?

Five a.m. was too early for a city-bred. But he'd been on the line by first light with the rest of them. She'd been right. It was hard work. The hardest he'd ever experienced . . .

Ben groaned and released his grip on the
steering wheel and shook his head to clear it. The
sun had long since slid into the Pacific and the cabin
was silhouetted against the darkening sky. He
shivered. Stiff from the long drive he eased himself
out of the Land Rover and packed his gear into the
cabin. At first he didn't think he was hungry, but
was soon grilling the halibut filet he'd picked up in
Malibu. That and a tossed salad quickly satisfied him
and he moved around the cabin, looking, touching,
remembering . . .

Ben knew that his father wanted him to
become a businessman like himself, but that was not
the kind of life he wanted for himself. The day after
his first semester at Pepperdine Ben told his father
his plans.

"I appreciate what you've done for me, Dad.
But business courses just aren't my thing. I want to
travel and write."

"Write? You can't make a living at that."

"I'm going to try."

Cecil Rush hadn't been happy with his son's
decision, but in the end he sighed. "Well, go ahead,
give it a go."

The first summer out of high school Ben had
gotten his seaman papers and sailed on coastwise
tankers for a year. That was enough of the sea, at
least as an ordinary seaman, so he'd enrolled at
Pepperdine, and majored in Journalism. He had met
Anne between his junior and senior years.

There had been little opportunity for pleasure
that summer in McCall. True to Anne's prediction,
fires were everywhere. He had slogged it out, often
fifteen or sixteen hours at a stretch, for the entire
summer. Once he'd had a two-day R & R in Boise,
and asked Anne to go with him.

She smiled shyly, color rising to her cheeks. She shook her head. "Sorry . . . I can't. Not this time."

On his last day in McCall, he'd stopped in the office. "I'm on my way home today. Catching a bus . . ."

"Oh." She sounded disappointed.

"How about lunch before I go?"

Her face brightened. "Okay. I'd love to. Give me five minutes."

That was their first and only date, if it could be called a date, all summer. But something happened to both of them that day that determined their future together. They walked to a small, crowded and noisy fast-food restaurant.

After they ordered, Ben found himself suddenly shy. Her hair had grown longer these past two months, and she had caught it behind with a green bow that exactly matched the color of her eyes. Usually he had no difficulty talking with women. But in ways that he couldn't quite put his finger on, Anne seemed to be different. A fragility of spirit. A searching quality in her eyes. A lostness, perhaps. Or a deep-seated aura of loneliness? Whatever it was, it drew him.

They talked in generalities about the fires, the summer. Then, heart pounding, he reached across the table and touched her hand. "Anne . . . I like you. May I write you, or telephone you, or something?"

She looked at him gravely and he marvelled at the depths of her eyes. Her response was one word, "Yes."

He abruptly changed the subject. "Why do you want to be a doctor?"

"I don't know. Maybe it has something to do with my mother and grandmother . . ."

She paused, a bird-like, ready-for-flight look in her eyes, as though she feared she had said too much. Awkwardly, Ben filled in the gap. "I'm going to be a writer."

"I know."

"How did you know?"

"You wrote it on your application."

He checked his watch and hoisted his bag to his shoulder. "Well, gotta go. Bus leaves in ten minutes . . ."

She jumped up too. "I'll walk to the depot with you." Just before he boarded, he impulsively bent and kissed her. He found a window seat and waved. She stood waving until the bus rounded the corner and was out of sight.

There were so many of her things in the cabin. Actually, it was more than a cabin, though they always referred to it as that. There were three bedrooms, only one of which they used as such. The other two had been turned into offices, one for each of them. Often, on long weekends, or for full weeks at a time, they would come here to read or to write, take long walks, make love, always relaxing each evening before the huge fireplace. Near the coast, and high as it was, the evenings were usually cool.

Anne's office was as she had left it: neat, orderly, everything in its proper place, her books and medical journals set in precise order on the shelves and in the cabinets. His was always a jumble of books, papers, magazine and newspaper clippings, the tools of his trade.

He walked into her room and opened a window, allowing the fresh mountain air to circulate and remove the stuffiness. He always felt somehow closer to her in this room than anywhere else, except for their bedroom where they had so often merged as one, in body and in mind.

A coyote howled and he heard an answering call from another hilltop. The whispering of the rising wind in the oleanders was a pleasant, companionable sound. He cocked his head to listen. He moved about, running his fingers across the bright-colored Navajo wool blanket on her divan. They had purchased it in Twin Wells, Arizona one summer where he had been researching a book on the Navajos. It had always been her favorite blanket, and she frequently wrapped herself in it as she worked at her desk.

Anne's books were for her, as his were for him, an extension of her being. Though she was an avid reader, and enjoyed occasional fiction, and biographies, she tended to read mostly medical journals and books. Just as she'd left them, a stack of new books and journals was beside her desk. A handful of frequently used books, *Dorland's Medical Dictionary*, the ever-present *PDR*, the *Physician's Desk Reference, Compendium of Drug Therapy*, and others, neatly lined up between the pair of pewter porpoise bookends he had given her on their first wedding anniversary.

He was dismayed to see the accumulated film of dust, which Anne would never have tolerated. He carefully removed the books from her desk one at a time and carried them to the open door to dust them. As he handled the PDR, a folded sheet of paper slid out and fell to the floor.

It was a handwritten note with three terse lines: "Anne, sorry to relay such distressing news by telephone. Cranston's workup is impeccable. He's a good man. I agree with him on every point, and remind you — as he did — that time is of the essence. Please begin therapy as soon as possible. Warm regards, Roland." The printed letterhead was from Roland Henson, M.D., Oncology. There was no date.

How long had she known before she had told him? he wondered, months? A year? Oh, God, why hadn't she shared her dread secret with him? He shivered, more from memories than from the chill.

But then, again, would it have made any difference if he had known? He balled his fist. It *might* have made a difference. By God, it *could have* made a difference! But then, who knows? She did, however, know so much more than he . . .

A gust of cool night air rustled the paper in his hand. He sighed and slid it back between the pages of the PDR where he'd found it and replaced the books. He noted that Anne's latest acquisitions — stacked neatly between her desk and divan — dealt primarily with homeopathy, acupuncture, nutrition and other alternative health modalities. She *had been* searching, seeking, hoping, praying . . .

He bent and read a few of the titles, some that had come after her death. Maybe he could pick up where she'd left off. He pulled a couple from the stack to begin reading.

Though he knew her so well, there was so much that he did not know. He felt robbed of the opportunity to have spent the rest of his life with her.

He turned off all the lights and stood at the front picture window. Far below he caught glimpses of Malibu-bound traffic on the coast highway. Miles away on the horizon he could make out a couple of freighters passing each other, one bound for Los Angeles, the other San Francisco, or further north. They had enjoyed watching the shipping lanes, and had never tired of speculating as to the cargoes and destinations of each ship.

Frequently Anne would whisper, ". . . like ships that pass in the night . . ."

Once she looked up at him meditatively. "Maybe that's us, Ben. Maybe we're like that, ships passing in the night."

He had started to chuckle, but the note of pathos in her voice prevented him. Instead, he nodded. "Could be . . ."

Chapter Two

In a dreamlike state, she seemed not to have heard him and softly began quoting from Tennyson, one of her favorite poets, "Sunset and evening star, And one clear call for me, And may there be no moaning of the bar, When I put out to sea. . . ."

She smiled up at him, and he was aware of a tear glistening on her cheek. Something in her expression forbade a response.

Finally, he undressed and slid between the cool sheets of their king-sized bed, luxuriating in the size of it, which was much larger than the smaller queen in their Santa Monica town house. But its very size, much too large for him alone, reminded him again of her absence. It seemed that everything he saw or touched reminded him of her.

Fingers clasped behind his head, gazing into the gloomy darkness that was not truly dark, he once again allowed the movies of his mind to spin reel after reel of memories of their lives together. As always, he was startled to note that the film never dimmed or faded. Each time they were as sharp, as bright, as clear as they had ever been.

CHAPTER THREE

She wasn't certain why, but she had been
unable to sleep that night. Benjamin Rush. Fresh and
clean looking. Ben Rush. The name sounded good to
her tongue. His application, which she had pulled
before she met him at the bus, told her he was six-
one. He must be all of that, she reasoned, because he
towered over her petite five-two. The photo he had
sent didn't do him justice. She snapped on her
reading light and sat up.

It was against regulations, she knew, but she
had removed his photo from the application and
brought it to her room. She held it away from her
and studied it. Brown curly hair, cut short. Nice
smile. Gentle, she thought. He had appeared to be
gentle. She hoped so. She was fearful of ungentle
people. She had always been afraid of loud speaking
and rough actions . . .

Like her father, with his courtroom, booming
voice that always hurt her ears. He frightened her.
She could never remember not being frightened of
him.

Her playroom at the Peak was huge, with toys
and books all around. So many that she was confused
by them all. She loved her oldest, raggediest teddy
bear, that was all coming apart at the seams. And
her soft, well-worn fabric *Velveteen Rabbit* book. The
others she played with when Nanny insisted.

"Here, Anne, play with this nice new dolly. Your daddy just bought it for you. Let me have the dirty old teddy bear . . ."

Nanny tried to pry the teddy bear from her three-year-old grasp, but Anne held on too tightly.

"No. No. I want my teddy bear. Don't want dolly."

When Daddy came and gave her a new toy, she would try to like it. Just to please him. But as soon as he went away, she refocused her attention upon her old, familiar, trustworthy favorites. They never made loud noises or changed. And never went away. Everything else in her world changed, or was noisy. Or went away. Except for her teddy bear and her *Velveteen Rabbit* book.

She could always depend upon them.

When she turned five, something irrevocable happened to her universe. Nothing was ever the same after that. Nanny woke her up and helped her bathe. "We must hurry, Anne . . . your breakfast is on a tray . . ."

"Why must I hurry?"

"Because you're going away . . ."

The fears that never left her intensified. "Going away? I don't want to go away. Where am I going?"

"You're going away to a nice school in the country."

She felt suddenly cold and frightened. "Are you coming with me, Nanny?"

Nanny laughed. "Of course not. You're a big girl now, Anne. Hurry, now. Johnson will be ready with the car. And we don't want to make him wait, do we?"

All the time she was talking, Nanny was dressing her. "What a nice, new dress you have, Anne. Aren't you happy to have so many new clothes?"

Anne shook her head. Everything she ever had was always new. The only thing she had that was old and soft and familiar was her worn, bedraggled teddy bear.

"I don't want to go away, Nanny. Will I come home tonight?"

"Don't be silly."

Johnson came to carry her little suitcase. Then he and Nanny led her down the huge spiral staircase, down to the marble foyer that Anne hated because it was so big and her voice echoed when she talked, and out to the big black car that drove Daddy to work. Only Daddy wasn't in the car. It was empty.

Johnson opened the door and held it. Nanny hugged her and said, "Get in, Anne. Have a nice time."

"Nanny, please don't make me go away. I want to stay here, with you. Please."

Nanny was very businesslike. "Anne, you *must* go. Your Daddy has made all the arrangements. He paid a lot of money . . ."

That always seemed to be the final argument: money. But it didn't mean anything to Anne. She had never had money and didn't even know what it was. But to big people, especially for Daddy and Nanny, money was *very* important.

She tried once again. "Please don't make me go."

Nanny smiled and gently but firmly pushed her into the open door of the black car. Not until that moment did Anne think of teddy bear. In a sudden panic she said, "But, I've got to have my teddy bear . . . I can't go without him . . ."

Nanny looked at Johnson and shook her head. "Mister Collins gave strict instructions. The teddy bear is not to go."

Anne suddenly felt so terribly alone. "Where is my Daddy? I want to tell him goodbye."

"He had to go to work early. He told me to tell you that he would write to you. And send you a new dress . . ."

In the end she finally went without seeing her Daddy, and without her teddy bear, or her *Velveteen Rabbit* book. She cried and cried, but Johnson didn't say anything, though she saw him look at her with his mirror. They drove for a long time until the car turned and drove through a pair of large black gates and stopped in front of a large brick building that had a lot of smaller brick buildings to the side.

Johnson opened the door and helped her out. "Well, here we are, Miss Anne."

She looked about at the wide grassy fields. She saw the high fence all around. And the gates. Why did everything have gates, she wondered. "But where are we?"

"This is your school."

He took her hand and led her up the wide concrete steps to the large double doors and took her inside . . . then he set down her suitcase and left without a word.

That was the first of many years of nights away from home in which Anne cried herself to sleep.

"Let her come and live with us," her grandmother Elias was saying. "Poor little tyke. She never knew her mother . . . and she's never known a mother's love . . ."

"I can take care of her," her father said. His voice sounded angry like it did when she had asked if the neighbor children could come to her toy room and play.

"She's not your responsibility, Magdalene. She's mine."

"But, Bertram, Anne *needs* a woman's care, a woman's love. I can give that to her."

"Magdalene, I've told you, Anne's got a Nanny. She's got a woman to care for her. That's all she needs."

Anne loved her grandmother's soft voice and wished her Daddy would let her live with Grandmother Elias. Even when speaking to her Daddy who always talked so awfully loud, Grandmother's voice was soft and kind.

"I know she has a Nanny, Bertram. I know that you provide for her. But it's not the same. Anne needs a woman . . . one of her own to love her."

"I'm in a hurry, Magdalene. I don't have time to go over this again. Anne's young. And resilient. She'll manage." Anne thought her father was about to shout again, like he shouted at Johnson and Nanny sometimes. She covered her ears with her hands.

Anne couldn't remember when she'd heard that conversation between her father and grandmother. Maybe she'd been three, or maybe four, she didn't know. But she thought about it often.

She had never known her mother. "She died when you were born," Nanny told her once. For days after that Anne was consumed with guilt that never completely went away. Her first remembrance of her father was of a cold, distant man, who never touched her. From as far back as she could remember, Anne tried desperately to attract his attention, to earn his love.

Even as an adult there always remained that part of her that was a little child, wondering what dreadful sin she had committed that her father could not love her. Her mind recognized him for what he was: a cold, grasping, ruthless man, but her heart simply could not learn the lesson.

No child could have tried harder than Anne. She was always at the head of her class, frequently the president. Still these strivings — and the victories — when they came, passed by her father unnoticed. Only when she failed to be first in anything did he make mention of her at all. He never came to her recitals, programs or graduations, and each absence became a new rejection of herself as a person, a new wound that refused to heal.

Once when she was quite young and was home for a holiday from the boarding school, she timidly approached him. "Daddy, can I go live with Grandmother? For just a little while?"

He puffed harder at his cigar and made the blue smoke go in big clouds around his head. "No, Anne. Don't ask me again. You will stay where I put you."

It was in gym class in her senior year in high school that Anne discovered the swollen lymph glands under her arms. She was terrified. She went home and sneaked copies of the *Merck Manual* and *Gray's Anatomy* from her father's extensive law and medical library and took them to her room. Fascinated, she read for hours on the subject.

Early the same year, Anne applied for and was accepted at Stanford, her father's alma mater. She was thrilled. Finally, she thought, I have done something that will please him. She rushed downstairs and knocked at his office door.

"Come in," he shouted gruffly, not bothering to look up from the legal brief he was working on. She stood before his desk uncertain of what to do.

"Yes, Anne. I know you are here. What is it now?"

"Daddy, I've been accepted at Stanford . . ."

"I expected you to be. Close the door on the way out."

She was crushed to the earth and was depressed for days. Once again she had failed to win his approval. What would it take?

Anne caught sight of Ben the next morning just before he climbed on board the truck with the other men. He was big and so handsome. He looked lean and trim in his work clothes. She wished she could wish him a good day. But it was too early and she hadn't dressed yet. She wondered what it would be like to have someone like Ben, someone who loved you, and who didn't shout at you, to love you and take care of you always . . .

A dozen fires were reported that day, and desperate calls went out for more men. She was on the phone all day. "Send more smoke jumpers! More trucks! More water drops! More supplies!"

Long before night she was weary to the bone, but there was more yet to be done. The ambulance brought burned and wounded men from the fire line. Each time she saw it she thought her heart would stop. The reports all went through her and she was relieved when Ben's name was not on the lists of injured.

Somehow the days dragged by.

Once she thought she saw him coming to the office, but it had turned out to be someone else. She never saw him to speak to, until several weeks had passed.

She was on the telephone that day when someone entered the office. She finished and turned around.

"Hi, Anne."

It was Ben. He was thinner. Browner. His curly hair needed trimming. He wore sharp-pressed khakis and a striped brown shirt, open at the front. When he smiled, she noticed how his eyes crinkled at the corner.

She put her hand to her throat, a purely reflex action. "Oh . . . hello, Ben."

"Uh, Anne, I've got a couple of days of R & R. Thought I'd go to Boise. See a movie or two . . ."

"That's nice," she said, wondering how her hair looked, wishing she'd worn a skirt instead of jeans.

"And I was wondering if you could go with me . . ."

Her heart fluttered. Oh, how I'd like to go with you, to Boise. Or anywhere. But she shook her head.

She could tell he was disappointed, but he smiled. "Well, my ride is about to leave. See you . . ."

He waved and was gone. And the brief sunlight of her day went with him. Why hadn't she gone? She had time coming. She could have gone. But the office was shorthanded. Would he ever ask her again?

That night she dreamed that recurrent dream of the mother she had never known . . .

Her eyes were closed and she was lying on something soft and warm and wonderfully comfortable. She could tell that it wasn't quite light, nor was it dark. Just in between. A sweet voice was singing to her. She couldn't quite hear the words, but they were peaceful words, loving words.

The voice stopped singing and spoke her name. "Anne . . . Anne. Are you awake?"

She was almost afraid to open her eyes for fear the voice and the warm safe feeling might go away. "Anne . . . Anne . . . I love you . . . I love you . . ."

She felt her muscles relax and she began to sink down deep into whatever it was she was lying on. Or in. She couldn't tell which. But it didn't matter. Whatever it was, it was wonderful. She was wrapped loosely in its folds, so loosely she knew she could extricate herself if she so desired.

"Anne . . . oh, Anne . . ." The voice was warm and soft. And all the fears she had felt when she was awake were chased away.

Ever so carefully, she opened her eyes.

And saw her mother.

Just like her picture. Long auburn hair. Green, green eyes. Maybe if she didn't open her eyes all the way her mother wouldn't go away. She closed her eyes. And that was when it happened. The gentle touch. On her hair . . . her face . . .

Suddenly a door slammed and the light went away.

Noises came. People shouting. Darkness.

And the gentle touch was gone . . .

"Anne . . . it's your grandfather . . ." His always strong voice had a quaver in it.

"Hello, Grandfather. Are you in Boise? Coming to see your fire-fighting granddaughter?"

"I wish that were so, Anne. But, no, I'm back home at Nob Hill. I just want to talk to you a minute. Is this a good time?"

Actually it wasn't a good time. The office was jammed with new applicants. The ambulance was due from the fire front just any minute. A new fire had just broken out across the lake. But, there was *something* in his voice . . .

"Yes, Grandfather, as good a time as any."

"It's about your grandmother . . . Magdalene . . ."

Anne felt a giant fist squeeze her heart. She struggled to breathe. "Grandmother? What do you mean?"

"She hadn't been feeling too well. You knew that . . ."

"Yes, I knew."

"Well . . ." she could tell he was crying. "Anyway . . . I finally got her to the doctor. And, it's . . . Anne, Honey . . . your grandmother's very sick . . ."

"What is it? What does the doctor say?"

"He called it lymphoma. Do you know what that is, Anne?"

"Yes, Grandfather, I know. Yes, I know." She felt a pain deep within her own body. "How . . . how bad is she? Is she at home? Is she in pain?"

"She's home now. And the doctor has given her something for the pain . . . but, she's not well. She wants to see you . . ."

Anne gripped the phone till her hand hurt. "Did he . . . did he say how much time?"

"No . . . except, a year or two. Maybe longer. Maybe less. He just couldn't say."

"Grandfather, I'm due to come home the first of the week. To register for the fall quarter. That's only four or five more days. Is that . . . will that be okay? I mean it would be awfully difficult to leave before that."

"Anne, that will be just fine. She'll be so happy to see you. So will I. Thank you, dear. I'll say goodbye for now. I love you. And Magdalene sends her love."

She sat still for several minutes, holding the dead phone in her hand, hardly aware of the crowded little office. Oh, God, no! Not Grandmother. The dearest person in all the world. *Not her*!

She worked mechanically, doing the things that had to be done, a film of tears in her eyes. She had to talk to someone. But who? Ben? No, he had gone back to Malibu a week ago. It warmed her a little just to think of those minutes with him the day he left: their lunch together, walking to the bus with him, then waving to him until the bus was out of sight.

Afterwards she realized she hadn't given him her address or telephone number. How would he ever write her or telephone her?

But maybe he hadn't meant what he had said anyway. Maybe he'd been just a dream . . . and nothing else.

The rest of the week was a blur. The goodbyes from the men. The bus to Boise. The flight to San Francisco. And the tearful visit at Nob Hill . . .

Then, back to Stanford. How could she possibly concentrate enough to attend classes? Somehow she must. If only she were a doctor now . . . maybe she could do something. Oh, God, help me. Help my dear, dear grandmother. I wish I could talk to Ben.

She hadn't reckoned with Ben's resourcefulness. He simply telephoned Stanford School of Medicine. "I'm one of Anne Collins' relatives," he told the Dean's secretary (under his breath he was saying, *I hope I soon will be related, closely related*), "and I must contact her . . ."

Moments later the telephone rang in Anne's room.

"Anne . . ."

She recognized his voice instantly. "Ben . . . I was afraid."

"Afraid of what?"

"That I might never hear from you again . . ."

He laughed and she remembered the way his eyes crinkled at the corners. "Not a chance. Not a chance."

"Where are you?"

"I flew up to San Francisco for the weekend. Hoping . . . just hoping that I could entice you to meet with me."

"Yes, I will meet you. Just tell me where . . ."

September 25 — Gross Anatomy again. I had nearly forgotten the terrible, almost unbearable smell. I could never become a surgeon: To take a scalpel in hand and actually slice into the living tissue of a living human body would be more than I could bear. My team has been given the cadaver of a man who died of, of all things, lymphoma. All I could think of was Grandmother Elias. Now I know why they call it "gross anatomy."

But I will persist. There must be something that can be done about that horrendous disease that's trying to take my sweet grandmother from me. If it is possible to find a way, I promise I will seek until I find it.

Ben called this evening. I will meet him in San Francisco on Sunday. I can hardly wait. I only hope I can soak or scrub away that awful formaldehyde smell before then!

How good it was to see him. How strong he looked. Not until this moment did she comprehend the depth of her need for him. He kissed her and she burst into tears.

"Why, Anne . . ." he said and wrapped his long arms around her.

"My whole world is coming apart . . ."

"Maybe I can help put it back together again."

She poured out her heart and he listened gravely, as she knew he would, holding her hands all the time. Somehow, just telling him made her feel better. Now she could handle it. Now she could be strong for Grandfather. And for Grandmother. She finished talking and he wiped away her tears.

"Now, dearest Anne, *Doctor Anne* . . . say, I *like* the sound of that. Let's do some fun things and forget for a while . . ."

Hand in hand, they walked along Fisherman's Wharf. Suddenly Anne began to laugh. And couldn't stop. She laughed until her sides hurt. Ben looked at her mystified.

Finally, tears running down her cheeks, she said, "I'm so very *glad* you brought me down here."

"Why? What's so funny? I don't get it."

She leaned toward him. "Smell my hair . . ."

He sniffed, still looking mystified. "Maybe I'm dense . . ."

"Ben, it's wonderful, the strong smell of fish. Now you can't smell that awful embalming stuff they put on the cadavers I've been dissecting."

They did the tourist things: rode the cable cars, ate in Chinatown, climbed Coit Tower. When Ben suggested Alcatraz, Anne shook her head. "No, Ben. Please, no. Prisons depress me. Let's go to happy places and do happy things."

November 20 — My clothes, skin and hair smell like death. I smell cadavers all day. I dream of them at night. I can rattle off "epidermis, dermis, subcutaneous fascia, deep fascia . . ." and so on in my sleep. The names of nerves and bones are becoming engraved into the very cells of my brain! All this is necessary, I know. We are studying the dead. When will we study the living? Do we have to understand dead tissue before we can understand living tissue? What does all this death have to do with healing?

Ben and I will be together for Christmas! Grandmother Elias has invited us to spend the holiday season with them at Nob Hill. She is feeling good enough to celebrate. They want to meet him. They will love him, I know. He is so filled with the joy of life that just being with him frees me for a time from my fear of disease and death.

Oh, what a paradox: I so want to live. But I have been alone and afraid so much that I am almost afraid to believe that Ben's love may help set me free.

As usual, the Elias' Nob Hill holiday decorations were a work of art. From within and without the century-old mansion, the lights of joy and peace radiated the love that was so much a part of Phineas and Magdalene themselves.

Anne was right. The Eliases *did* love Ben. It was a case of mutual love at first sight.

Dinner with a carefully-selected list of the most intimate friends, followed by a time of music around the massive Steinbeck that graced one corner of the dark-panelled living room.

Phineas himself, his lined face wreathed in smiles, distributed gifts to his guests. Sitting beside Anne who contentedly leaned against him, Ben indicated the mantlepiece.

He whispered, "Isn't that a menorah?"

"Yes . . . it's a Marc Chagall . . . from Jerusalem."

"But, why does it have *nine* candles instead of seven?"

"The *seven*-candled menorah is the traditional symbol of Judaism. The Hanukkah menorah that you see, is an eight-branched candelabrum. The highest candle is called the shammash, and is used to light all the others. Tonight is the eighth night of Hanukkah. That's why all of the candles are lit."

"Then your grandparents are Jewish?"

"Of course. Does it matter?"

"No, not really. Actually, not at all."

Anne squeezed his hand. "Do you like them, my grandparents?"

"Yes . . . they are lovely people."

"They like you, too, Ben. And that makes me happy."

Ben's presence in her life helped quell some of the ever-present fears of imminent disaster that had plagued her all her life. But even he could not eradicate the fear of the insidious monster that was stealing away the life of her grandmother, the kindest woman she had known in her limited world.

"Hello, Father," she said when Bertram finally returned the call she had placed earlier in the day.

"Anne, I'm very busy. What is it you want?"

"I just wondered if you knew about Grandmother Elias. She's been very ill . . ."

"Yes, Anne, I know. She's got cancer."

His response was a cruel rebuff and she felt hurt and empty again, sorry she had tried to communicate with him. "Oh . . ." she stammered, "I thought you might not know . . . and . . ."

"Is that all, Anne? Do you need more money?"

"That's all, Daddy. I guess I don't need anything. Thank you." It was a lie. She *did* need something. Something she was yet unable to acknowledge that her father could never provide.

She hung up the phone slowly . . .

Anne looked again at her grandparents' picture above her desk, next to one of her mother taken a few months before her death. Turning her desk lamp up as bright as it would go, Anne studied carefully the faces of the two women. As always, she was amazed by her own striking resemblance to Magdalene Elias. Except that she had inherited her mother's distinctive emerald-green eyes . . .

CHAPTER FOUR

Ensconced in the high-backed leather chair of his opulent, mahogany-panelled office comprising the entire ground-level north wing of his nineteenth-century Twin Peaks mansion, Bertram Collins resembled nothing so much as a huge brown bear. So much so that his opponents and detractors referred to him as Ol' Grizzly. And his obvious success in his litigious world had earned him the somewhat begrudging title of Grizzly King.

"Let them call me what they want to," Collins said on more than one occasion. "But I'm the legal king of this city, *and* this state. And they all know it."

Son of an immigrant shipyard worker, Bert determined early that he would make something of himself. That determination, he often bragged, stemmed from the time when he heard his fourth grade teacher refer to him as "that Collins wharf rat." Furious, Bert had plotted his revenge. He learned where the teacher lived, then devised retribution worthy of the crime. He trapped a dozen large wharf rats and loosed them in the teacher's home late one night. She never called Bert a "wharf rat" again.

The Collins family lived in the small community of Brisbane, a suburb of San Francisco, and Alex Collins was a pipe fitter at Newcastle Steel Shipyards at Hunter's Point. He was a steady worker, but except for the newspaper and union propaganda, he seldom read anything. Bert considered his father dull and boring, and vowed to become as unlike him as possible. He discovered the incredible world of books by the age of seven, and from that time on, the library was his escape route from his squalid existence. He loved reading about pirates and Indian fighters. But he finally settled upon Jesse James as his hero. It was from Jesse James' philosophy that Bert formulated his own: "Cause a person to fear you and you'll master him."

Hungry for power, Bert sought it wherever it was, or where it appeared to be. In his early teens, street gangs seemed to offer the best route. He became as rough as the roughest. But he saw too many of his gang members killed in gang skirmishes, or busted and sent to prison, so he realized the futility of that road to fame. After much thought, Bert knew education held the key to his future.

Typically, he plunged in with all his might, and by diligent effort Bert finished high school at age 16, then applied and was accepted at Stanford. Finally, he told himself, I'm on the right track. He had no illusions concerning the difficulties he would face, but rightly or wrongly, he had seen the power of the law. He would become a lawyer, a rich and powerful lawyer. It was a miracle he survived the struggle. He expected and received no financial assistance from his father. But Alex did what he could: he got Bert a job in the shipyards, on the night shift.

The work was hard and dirty, but he could work nights and go to school during the day. Often he would sleep only three or four hours in twenty four. He made it a practice *never* to go to class unprepared. Only once did he fail this promise to himself, and then only when he was injured on the job and forced to spend the night in the hospital.

He lost weight and became thin and hollow-eyed from lack of sleep and proper food. But he vowed he would make it, and bent all his powers to that goal. He was a man possessed. A tribute to his ruthless struggle to succeed is the fact that he was able to make Law Review in his final year. Nothing, he promised himself, nothing or nobody will ever stand in my way.

The young man was canny enough to know that a degree was one thing, but even with a law degree from Stanford you had to have connections. He had no connections. Connections meant money. And money meant referrals from the right people. But how? He didn't know, but he knew there *must be* a way.

Somehow, he knew, he had to tap the rich resources of San Francisco's elite. And how better to do that than through a woman. A woman whose father held the reins of power. He would find that woman. He would find her, woo her, win her and use her as his ticket, his passage to the Other Side.

Books he knew. The library he knew. These had been his tools since he was a small boy. The goal: Find a rich and powerful man with an unmarried daughter. Scorning even the little sleep he had been getting, he began devouring the society columns. Time and again he would locate the right family, the right woman, only to read of her betrothal a few weeks later.

That lead him to the formula. Simple but effective: Those society women who caught their men were lovely, the pick of the city. Which meant the opposite must also be true. The not-quite-so-lovely ones did not always get their men.

He would best them at their game. Instead of the hunted, he would become the hunter. He would hunt and he would capture the richest one of them all. The one whose very lack of physical loveliness had failed to net the most eligible men. He labored under no false concepts of his own physiognomy. He *knew* he was not handsome. He *knew* that he had no connections. But he also *knew* that he could win what he set out to win.

One name finally surfaced that met all his qualifications: the only daughter of the rich and powerful Phineas Elias. The name Elias he knew, for it frequently appeared in the papers, along with other socially prominent people of means. It was a rare find. The Elias family was one of the original old-money people that traced their beginnings — and their wealth — back to the very roots of California, even San Francisco itself.

Beatrice was the only child of Phineas and Magdalene Elias. They wanted more children to help fill their Nob Hill mansion, but Magdalene did not succeed in becoming pregnant again.

The Eliases doted on the child, pampering the tiny, red-headed girl to distraction. "What does it matter?" Magdalene said. "We love her and she knows we love her. Love, after all, is really all that matters."

Phineas agreed. "Yes. We have a healthy daughter who looks just like her father." Full of emotion, his voice wavered, "And I still have her mother. That is enough. *Baruch ha shem.*"

Bertram knew nothing of all this, nor would it have made a difference if he had. He read the account of Beatrice Elias' coming out ball. For his scheme, Beatrice Elias would fit the bill perfectly. To his calculating eye, the girl was not beautiful, hardly even attractive by his definition, but that was a mere detail. She possessed other, even more important qualifications: Namely, by right of heirship she was the access, the pipeline so to speak, to millions of very attractive dollars.

He began to stalk her as carefully as any hunter stalks his game.

Week after week, he read everything to be read of the City's elite. After her coming out ball, the girl's name was not once mentioned again. That could mean only one thing, he reasoned, Beatrice Elias had not as yet been spoken for.

Therefore, he reasoned, he, Bertram Collins, a very eligible bachelor, who was soon to pass his bar exam and become an attorney at law, he would find her. He would meet her. And he would win her, both her *and* her money.

He hired a private detective to determine Beatrice's social habits: where she frequently took dinner, her favorite places to shop, her days and places of leisure. Everything. And when he learned all there was to learn of Beatrice's peregrinations, he set the trap. On Monday Miss Beatrice Elias frequently dined alone at a tiny club on Geary Street. He coordinated his efforts to do the same.

He set the date — phoned for a reservation, dressed for the occasion, and went to dinner.

Promptly at eight, she arrived and took her place at her accustomed table. Just before she had given the waiter her order, he arose from his seat, walked over and bowed respectfully.

"Miss Elias, please do not think me forward, but allow me to introduce myself . . ." which he proceeded to do with all the social ease at his disposal. Having done that, he proceeded, "And since I, too, am dining alone, would you allow me the privilege of dining with you?"

As he anticipated, the direct approach worked. She looked him over carefully, noting his well-cut clothing, his impeccable manners (which he had learned to perfection), and smiled. "Yes, Mister Collins, I see no harm in that. Please join me . . ."

From that moment on, according to his well-rehearsed plan, he was in complete control. He was careful not to move too fast, nor too slowly. But it took only a few weeks before Beatrice invited him to the Elias's home for dinner. Phineas, of course, had Bertram carefully checked out, and had serious reservations about him from the report he received.

But Bert had played his cards right. Beatrice had fallen in love with him. As the only daughter, *and* the sole heir to the Elias fortunes, Beatrice was accustomed to having her own pampered way. She had always done it, now she exercised her learned prerogatives and did it again. When Elias exhibited less than enthusiasm over her choice, Beatrice took the bit in her teeth. And when Bert asked her to marry him, propitiously just a week after he had passed his bar examination, she said yes.

She had been intrigued by his quite obvious adulation of herself, along with his burning desire to achieve. He, on the other hand, was intrigued by her ancestry, the political power at her disposal (through her father), and their millions that were lying "moldering" (he thought) in several banks of California.

Phineas and Magdalene soon saw that they were outvoted and gave in as graciously as possible. Beatrice demanded, and got for herself and her intended groom, the wedding of the year. All the prominent of the City were present, and Bert was off and running. At a seemingly obtuse remark he made to Beatrice, who picked it up immediately, Bert's father-in-law set him up in an office on Market Street and referred a number of his social registry friends to his son-in-law. Bert very capably did the rest.

He parlayed that inauspicious beginning into a legal and political power to be reckoned with. Along the way, he picked up Lloyd Gould, a promising young attorney, and offered him a "full partnership" for a "reasonable figure," Lloyd's father was well able to afford. It proved to be yet another winning combination.

Then luck and opportunity played into his hands.

Lloyd Gould's young niece contracted polio as a result, the family averred, of the polio vaccine the girl was given two weeks before her fifth birthday. Bert

saw his golden opportunity and skillfully engineered
the opportunity for his fledgling company to represent
the girl's family. On their behalf, he accepted the case
on a contingency basis, and mounted a $25,000,000
class action suit against the vaccine drug company,
the clinic, the administering physician and nurse, and
as many as fifty John and/or Jane Does who
participated in the transaction.

So convincing was the brief Bert prepared that
the case never went to court. Fearing the adverse
publicity, the defendants quietly settled, making Bert
an overnight millionaire, and the most sought-after
litigator west of the Mississippi.

Collins' good fortune did not end there. The
week following his brilliant coup, he received a
telephone call from Roger Keller, Chairman of the
Board for Bullion Inc., International. Recognizing
Collins' clever and devious expertise, Bullion's Board
of Directors opted to have him on their side instead
of against them. Consequently Keller was authorized
to make Collins an offer he could not refuse. With
Collins' aggressive, self-seeking firm running
interference for them, BII would be virtually assured
a growing supremacy in the pharmaceutical market.

Keller laid his plans carefully. The Executive
Board had empowered Keller to offer Collins
"anything it takes to get him." Keller did not intend
to return home without his prey.

Collins' research had assured him that this
giant of the pharmaceutical industry had virtually
unlimited exchequer at their disposal. Beyond that,
Collins learned, BII's political and financial tentacles
extended into virtually every phase of the world's
gigantic health-care industry: hospitals, insurance
companies, medical associations and schools, and well-
placed stooges in government regulatory agencies.

With few questions asked, Bullion was willing
to barter dollars and position for Collins' genre of

legal skill. Though dollars were important to Collins, he was ready to sell his soul for power.

The meeting between the two was classic. Keller suggested The Big Four at The Huntington on Nob Hill. Collins agreed, but personally made the reservation: a quiet corner where Keller would have to squint to look at him. Altogether, each man had studied and stalked his quarry with patience and skill.

Face to face with Bertram Collins, Roger Keller's gut instinct told him Collins was their man. If ever he beheld the piranha, killer instinct in a man, he saw it in Collins' deeply-inset brown eyes that chilled him with their glow of cool, detached, ruthless cunning. Peering at the man over the edge of his martini glass, Keller watched Collins read Bullion's financial report with an excitement he was barely able to conceal.

Seated across the table from Keller, Collins sensed the "winner-take-all" attitude that radiated from Bullion's Chairman of the Board. Instinctively he realized the price tag on this transaction was of little importance. The meeting of minds was primary. Inside himself he knew the victory was his.

With hardly any ado, Keller came to the point. "We have agreed in principle on the telephone," he said. He slid a one-page document across the table. "Now, let's see if we agree in fact . . ."

Despite his wildly-beating heart, Collins casually bit the end from his cigar, lit it and exhaled a cloud of smoke before he reached for the contract. His well-trained legal mind took in the basics at a glance. He quickly skipped over the monetary figures. They, he knew, were negotiable. He was looking for something else. To his absolute delight, it was all there, in bold print. The man who signed this agreement, Collins saw, would be installed as legal watch dog over Bullion's health care interests —

buttressed by the wealth and political backing of one of the world's pharmaceutical giants.

In a word: nigh unlimited *power*.

Collins looked up. "That's it?"

Keller nodded. "That's it."

Collins reached for his pen. "Need a witness?"

"No witness necessary."

Collins signed one copy and kept the duplicate. Keller slid another envelope across the table. Without opening it, Collins pocketed it. "Anything else?"

"No. That does it."

"Any special instructions?"

"We'll be in touch."

"Good. I've got to get back to my office."

"And I've got a plane to catch."

They shook hands and parted. The meeting had taken a scant thirty minutes.

Bert immediately sought property worthy of himself. He found a huge estate on Twin Peaks that was being sold for taxes. With a large portion of his recently acquired fortune, he set about restoring the old property to its former glory. A year and substantial dollars later, when the project was completed, Collins greased the proper political wheels and had "The Peak House" — as he chose to name it — designated as an historical landmark and tourist attraction.

Bert was having the time of his life. Such was not the case with Beatrice. She awoke from her romantic reverie to find herself not only pregnant, but relegated to the most miserable existence she could ever imagine. It didn't take too many months for her to realized that she had been used, and that she was a mere pawn in Bertram's larger game of chess. To state that her marriage was loveless would be to beg the question.

She was ashamed and very much alone. How could she now go to her loving parents and admit to her terrible mistake. Though the Eliases suspected such, Beatrice tried to conceal the enormity of the error of her ways.

When she tried to appeal to Bertram, he merely laughed. "I know I married you. That was merely a formality, a convenience. I'm *really* married my profession. And a man can have only one mistress . . ."

Whether or not Bertram Collins truly loved that mistress was open to conjecture. He did, however, love the power, prestige and wealth she brought him, in approximately that order. In exchange she demanded of him his total time and attention, which he willingly gave, not even allowing himself the doubtful pleasure of taking a vacation, which he was never known to do.

Bertram was seldom home and when he was, he seemed hardly to be aware of her existence. Beatrice's pregnancy was difficult and her labor worse. When it came time for her to deliver, Bertram was also delivering — a speech in Boston. His was accompanied by greater applause than hers. After more than 48 hours of hard labor, when Beatrice had gone beyond her strength, the baby girl had to be taken by cesarean.

The baby survived. The mother did not.

Bert didn't mourn Beatrice'sdeath, because he had never loved her. She had been merely a convenience, a figurehead, a symbol of his leap from poverty and obscurity to prominence and power; and the leash that held Phineas in check as Bert climbed the ladder of social and financial success.

The baby was both an inconvenience and a pawn, a hostage. Phineas and Magdalene longed to raise their granddaughter, but Bertram's paranoia led him to believe they would undermine his control, so he rejected their request. Instead, he hired a series of nannies to care for Anne, then generally dismissed the child from his mind.

CHAPTER FIVE

The ceremony that transformed the neophytes into full-fledged bona-fide doctors took place on a bright, clear afternoon in June. Phineas and Magdalene were there. Ben, who had flown up in the morning and would take the red-eye back to LA late that night, was there. Bertram Collins, who had never before found it convenient to grace any of Anne's previous notable events with his presence, but who was an honored guest at this one, was also present. Anne was euphoric.

After the preliminary, mostly self-congratulatory speeches, including Bertram Collins, and announcements had been made and were out of the way, Dean Charles arose in all his pomp and splendor, looking for all the world like a high priest in his crimson robes, which was, of course, the idea, and instructed the students to rise and repeat after him the ancient physician's Credo — the Hippocratic Oath.

Anne Collins, along with all the assembled metamorphosing students, responded to the solemnity of the occasion. Hardly a parent, family member or fend of the graduates moved or even squirmed, as the students repeated the mystical words.

I swear by Apollo the physician to hold my teacher in this art equal to my own parents . . .

Dr. Anne's Journal

Equal to my own parents? Anne wondered, in confusion. To do everything for one's own benefit, as my father does, instead of for the benefit of others?

To consider his family as my own brothers and to teach them this art . . . without payment . . .

Without payment? How can this be sworn to? When most of my colleagues speak of little else than being enriched by their chosen profession. And I, myself, are my motives pure and above reproach in this regard?

I will use my best judgment to help the sick and do no harm . . .

Do no harm? Anne stumbled over the words. Statistically, she had just learned, that a *minimum* of 40% of all tonsillectomies and hysterectomies performed annually in the U.S. are known to have been unnecessary. And that 78,000 people get cancer from X-rays each year. Do no harm?[1]

I will not give any fatal drugs to anyone — even if I am asked. Nor will I suggest any such thing . . .

What about chemotherapy? Anne had read of the low success rate of such therapy, and how it often caused irreversible damage to the brain central nervous system, even death.[2] [3] What about the 1955 epidemic of polio traced to incorrectly prepared vaccine? Or the 2.6 million expectant mothers caused to miscarry because of the highly-touted drug DES?[4]

Nor will I give a woman a pessary to procure abortion . . .

A "pessary," Anne knew from discussion of this part of the Credo, was a device inserted in the vagina to treat uterine prolapse, uterine retroversion, or cervical incompetence. A diaphragm pessary, she knew, was also used for contraception. All of which seemed to be beside the point. The point of it all, she thought, was that the Oath appeared to be ethically opposed to abortions for any reason. Were abortions never to be performed under *any* circumstances?

56

What about rape or incest or emotional instability? What about a woman's right to control her own body? Were there to be *no* exceptions to this blanket vow?

I will be chaste and religious in my life and in my practice . . . I will not use the knife, not even to remove the stones within . . .

Chaste and religious, yes. But, what about surgery? Anne remembered the debates she and other students had had over the benefits versus the hazards of surgery.

I will not abuse my authority to indulge in sexual contact. I will never divulge the secrets of my patients, regarding them as holy . . .

Dean Charles' rich bass voice paused. A deep hush settled over the vast assemblage. It seemed that his eyes met and held for a moment the eyes of every student, one at a time. He took a deep breath and pronounced the benediction . . .

"Ladies and gentlemen . . . you are now physicians. Go from this place and do honor to your chosen profession."

Nothing, Anne realized, nothing that I have ever done or felt can possibly match this experience. A spontaneous sob shook her small frame. "I have made a commitment," she whispered to nobody in particular, "a commitment to serve humanity with all the healing knowledge at my disposal. And I shall never violate that commitment. So help me, God."

Ben had made reservations for hors d'oeuvres and dessert at the Top of the Mark Hopkins, where from that exalted height, with the panorama of San Francisco Bay spread out before them, and the amber lights of the Oakland Bay Bridge blinking a welcome through the fog, Ben touched his glass to Anne's and proposed a toast.

"To the lovely *Doctor* Anne, whom I shall always cherish."

"Oh, Ben, how nice."

He slid the little box across the table. "Open it."

The diamond sparkled in the candlelight, highlighting the green of her eyes. Despite himself, Ben's heart skipped a beat. "Oh, Ben, it's beautiful. I love it!"

He beamed. "Anne, I've loved you since the day I saw you in McCall with the spot of soot on your cheek. And I herewith am *formally* asking you to marry me . . ."

She stretched out her left hand and admired the ring. Her eyes glittered with unshed tears. "Oh, Ben . . . yes."

He nearly toppled his wine glass when he leaned across the table to kiss her. "I've never been so happy in my life."

It had been many years since Anne had tried to have a meaningful conversation with her father. And, the Sunday morning after Ben's proposal, she hoped would be the day when this would occur. She timed her arrival at breakfast to coincide with his. Before entering the morning room that caught the sun as it rose across the Bay, and where Lucy served breakfast, Anne paused to quiet her pounding heart, fix a frightened smile upon her face before she entered.

Bertram, his huge bulk squeezed into a red and yellow sport shirt and shorts, overflowing his chair, was squinting at the *Examiner*. He gulped down a huge bite of toast, bent a corner of the paper so he could peer over it, and rumbled, "Well, do I address you as *Doctor* now? Or is Anne still okay?"

"Daddy! I'll always be Anne to you."

He cleared his throat, grunted what was meant to sound like, "Congratulations," and started to retreat behind his paper.

"Wait, Daddy, I have an announcement."

He paused with his paper at half mast. "Announcement?"

"Ben proposed last night. I accepted. We're to be married on July 15th. Here, at the Peak . . ." The words came out in a burst of energy, as though she knew she must get them out before she lost her nerve.

Bertram's paper remained in fixed position. He didn't blink, further unnerving his already nervous daughter.

"At least, I'd *like to be* married here. That is, if it would be all right with you."

Her voice trailed off, ending with a weak, "Please?"

"You'll have your wedding here. And I'll handle all the arrangements." With those words, Bertram's eyes turned back to the *Examiner*. The conversation was over.

Collins outdid himself to make Anne's wedding a lavish event, the San Francisco social highlight of the year. But Anne felt like she was on the outside looking in, merely a spectator in what was to have been *her* day. True to his word and true to form, Bertram did handle all the arrangements, leaving Anne feeling uninvolved and more unloved than before. He did again what he had so often done before: utilize a social event to achieve a business gain.

July 25 — Ben says honeymoons can last forever, but my first day (actually 24 hours) at Santa Monica's St. Luke Hospital. Perhaps it's because of my grandmother, but I seem to be obsessed with cancer. I see it all about me. Why is cancer increasing so fast? Had former President Nixon's proclaimed "war on cancer" been only a political maneuver?

Dr. Anne's Journal

Are we, as the New England Journal of Medicine stated, ". . . losing the war against cancer"?[5] I shudder to think of our country's future.

"I've been assigned to Oncology," Anne told Ben, "the most depressing department of the entire hospital. I am beginning to believe that cancer is the scourge of mankind."

"Maybe you can help change that."

"How can that be when billions are being spent on research — with so little to show for it?"

"Maybe," Ben responded darkly, "maybe they're on the wrong trail. Maybe they're all looking in the wrong place for the answer."

"What do you mean by that?"

"I'm not really sure what I mean. Except that it seems to me that everybody's looking for a cancer *cure*, when they can't even agree on what it is or what causes it."

Anne was to consider Ben's answer for a long time.

When Anne began her internship, Ben settled into his writing routine. He set up his IBM computer in their spare bedroom, built bookcases along one whole wall, and dragged out the notes for the novel he had been dreaming of writing.

Anne's unpredictable, often super-long hours made cooking and housework impossible chores for her to handle. Ben did for her what she couldn't do for herself. And when she dragged her weary body home after her sixteen, twenty, and often twenty-four hour shifts, she found that he'd cheerfully kept the home fires burning.

"I think my mind's turning to stale oatmeal," she told him one morning.

"You'll make it, Doctor Anne," he affirmed, as he massaged her cramping back and leg muscles so she could sleep.

"I know *I'll* make it," she groaned, "but will all of my patients make it?"

"Of course they will."

"I'm not always so sure . . . because . . ." The sentence was never completed. Anne had fallen asleep.

"I'm being rotated to ER, Emergency Room," Anne announced one night. "I don't think I'll like that . . ."

"Good experience, though," Ben commented.

"Perhaps. But not the *kind* of experience I want to have."

"What kind do you want?"

"In two words: cancer research. But not the remote, isolated kind of research that's usually associated with laboratories. I want to work with people who are sick — people with cancer — and help them to get well. I want to take time to know them. To find out why they are sick, to find out the *causes* behind their illnesses. And then work on removing the causes instead of treating the results . . ."

"To paraphrase," he grinned, "also, to coin a phrase, you don't like putting a Bandaid on a cancer."

"Exactly."

Anne's youthful appearance and petite size occasionally mitigated against her, and she was often mistaken for a candy striper, a fact that caused her constant irritation. One night she had just begun suturing a victim's knife wound when he cursed and jerked away from her. "Git outta here, woman!" he shouted. "Don't want no dumb nurse a'sewin' me up. Leave me be and git me a real doc!"

"I *am* a real doctor. Please lie still."

"You ain't no doc. You're jist a kid. Git away from me!"

She had to call for the resident to complete the job she had started. The resident berated the patient.

Dr. Anne's Journal

"You just missed your chance, buddy. Dr. Rush's the best seamstress around here. Now you've got to put up with me. Lie still now, before I give you a shot of something to knock you out!"

"You'all puttin' me on? Tryin' to tell me that dame's really a doc?"

"That's right. Now lie still!"

A pregnant young woman injured in a car accident was in labor when the ambulance brought her in. Almost before they got her loaded onto the gurney, her baby was crowning. Anne ran alongside the gurney as they wheeled the barely 16-year-old girl to Maternity.

"Help me, Nurse . . . please help me!" the girl screamed. "The baby's coming! Get me a doctor!"

"Just take it easy, lady," Anne soothed. "I'm a doctor. And you and your baby will be just fine . . ."

> *October 3 — One of the patients in my section committed suicide today. A white woman, 38 years old. Uterine cancer.*
> *She told me she had been ill for about four years. She said, "Doctors have done everything — surgery, four times; chemotherapy, three series; radiation, all of it. And I am not getting better. They know it and so do I. They tell me I've got to go through the whole procedure again, even though I don't want to."*
> *Mostly she's been fairly upbeat and cheerful. Yesterday she was depressed. She asked me to hold her hand and talk to her, which I did. During the night she slit her wrists and was dead when the nurse made her rounds.*

Anne was depressed for days.

Chapter Five

She saw Dr. Stephens, one of the oncologists, in the lunch room and asked him, "How many of your patients die?"

He shrugged, "Quite a few of them."

"What percentage?"

He gave her a harsh look. "You're new, aren't you?"

"Yes. I've been here just two or three months."

"You're asking too many questions that don't concern you," he grated between his teeth, and slammed out of the room.

During that year, due largely to the efforts of his agent, who recognized a novelist prodigy when he saw one, Ben's first novel had been snapped up by a major publisher. The generous advance would take care of their expenses for nearly a year.

As her internship drew to close, realizing that positions for young, inexperienced doctors were not easy to come by, Anne began making applications for a cancer research position. But a phone call one night changed the direction she was headed.

"Dr. Rush, please," a strange male voice said.

"This is Dr. Rush speaking."

"My name is Allen Drury. Dr. Allen Drury. Your father told me that you're about to complete your internship and that you are looking for a place to practice."

Anne groaned inwardly. Father is four hundred miles away, yet he's still holding a tight rein to my life. She drew a deep breath. "Yes, I will be completing my internship in less than two months."

She heard pages turning. "Oh, yes, here it is. Dr. Rush, I'll have a few minutes tomorrow afternoon, about five-fifteen. Could you stop by my office so I can show you around. And so we can talk?"

She struggled for control. Why does Father continue doing this to me? Surely not because he loves me. Then, why? Finally she did what she had always done. Knowing how angry he would be if she didn't accede to his demands, she gave in.

"Why, yes, Dr. Drury," she said. "Five-fifteen is a good time. I'll plan to be there."

"Thank you, Doctor. See you then. My address is . . ."

Ben looked up from the book he'd been reading. "Sounds like it could be important?"

"I suppose it could be. But I don't understand. Just exactly who is this Dr. Drury and how does he know my father?"

Allen Drury's office, on Wilshire Boulevard in Beverly Hills, Anne discovered, was a well-appointed, softly-lighted office suite. Tasteful, classical music completed the backdrop of quiet confidence that Drury evidently desired to project for his patients. Only one name, however, Allen Drury, M.D., was on the door, a fact that surprised her.

An attractive, platinum-blonde nurse Anne judged to be in her late twenties was seated at the reception desk, completing a telephone call when Anne arrived.

The young woman looked up and smiled. "May I help you?" Her voice, Anne noticed, was pleasantly throaty, melodious.

"I have an appointment with Dr. Drury at five-fifteen. I think I'm a trifle early. My name is Anne Rush."

"Oh, yes, Dr. Drury is expecting you." She arose and extended her hand in greeting. "I am Carolyn Kemp, Dr. Drury's nurse. If you'll make yourself comfortable, I'll tell Dr. Drury that you are here."

Carolyn rapped on a door down the hallway. At a muffled response, Carolyn opened the door and spoke to someone inside. Then she turned and beckoned.

Chapter Five

August 1 — This is my first day ta
practice with Dr. Allen Drury. Dr. Drury
says he is a friend of my father's, and
that my father specifically wanted me to
work with him. I'm not aware of their
relationship, but if it will please Father
for me to practice with Dr. Drury, I'll
give it a try. For a time, until I can get
involved in cancer research. I
understand that Dr. Jack Drury, Allen's
son had been practicing with his father
until just recently, when he left to open
his own office in East Los Angeles. I
gather there was some friction between
the two men over medical philosophy.

For the first time in their married life, even
with Anne's occasional early morning surgeries (she
had finally overcome her squeamishness to some
degree in that regard), the Rushes were now able to
settle into a more or less regular routine. By careful
management they built for themselves a getaway
cottage — which they affectionately referred to as
"our cabin" — in the rugged coastal hills above
Malibu.

To traverse the somewhat rugged "trail"
between Pacific Coast Highway (the "locals" called it
PCH) and their cabin, Ben splurged and purchased a
somewhat battered Land Rover he'd been eyeing for
several months. The Rover proved to be an excellent
vehicle for their somewhat irregular trips.

Except for occasional professional conventions,
the Rushes had few social responsibilities or
engagements. Though pressured at times by deadlines
and schedules, their home life, indeed, their total
situation, was quite placid and almost idyllic.

The only real flaw of which they were aware
was Magdalene's condition, which, though currently
stable, presented a rather uncertain prognosis.

Dr. Anne's Journal

Evenings Ben generally reserved for light reading, which Anne utilized to keep up on her medical literature. She, even more than Ben, had a nightly ritual from which she rarely deviated. After her rejuvenating soak in the tub, she would note the day's events in her Journal.

Anne considered those regular entries a serious commitment. To what or to whom she wasn't sure. But, from that first notation in med school, which she had initiated at the suggestion of a professor, she seldom missed. Though that had been her reason for beginning, even Anne herself, as she once admitted to Ben, could not clearly articulate her reasons for continuing.

"I only know that it's important," she said, "at least it's important to me."

"Maybe it's become a diary of our marriage?" Ben teased.

"Perhaps."

"May I read it?"

"Of course."

"When?"

"Any time. Now, if you'd like." She tossed it to him.

Ben leafed through a few pages, handing it back with a grin. "Diary, Dr. Anne? That's not a diary. It's a medical treatise."

"I'm glad you concur. That's what it's supposed to be."

"One day I'll read the whole thing," Ben said, little realizing the prophetic import of those words. Neither of them could possibly have known at that moment what a vital place Anne's Journal would one day play in both their lives.

CHAPTER SIX

The light changed at Wilshire and Veteran, and the bright red, late model Mercedes convertible jumped ahead of the other vehicles, cut across three lanes of traffic and slid smoothly onto the Northbound 405. "This is KRFN, your Radio Freeway News . . ." the muted voice of the radio newsman spoke to the lone occupant, "bringing you up to the minute local and national news . . .

"In a surprise move today, Roger Keller, Chairman of the Board for BII, Bullion Inc., International, announced the takeover of two smaller domestic drug companies, thus becoming the largest pharmaceutical company in the United States. Legal maneuvers for the merger, Keller said, were provided by the prestigious San Francisco law firm, Collins, Gould, Razinski and Goldman, spearheaded by Bertram Collins, the firm's founder and senior partner. The move resulted in a flurry of activity on Wall Street . . ."

"He's done it again," Allen Drury said aloud. "He's got the nose of a bloodhound . . . and the Midas touch." He shook his head in wonderment and snapped off the radio as he maneuvered the Mercedes smoothly through the fast-moving traffic to exit on Mulholland. "But then, he always has . . ."

There were five of them shivering in the gloom of the old warehouse. None was past his mid-teens;

all were dressed poorly in a conglomerate mixture of sweaters, castoff Navy pea coats and old jackets. Three wore black stocking caps pulled down over their ears. The others were hatless and alternately rubbed their red, chapped hands and cupped them over their ears. They muttered amongst themselves as they passed the joint around.

"He's late," the smallest of them said harshly. "He's always late . . . I don't think he's coming."

"He'll be here."

"What makes you so sure?"

"Cause he *said* he'd be here."

"Think he'll deliver?"

"He always does, doesn't he?"

"Yeah . . . yeah, he does. But it's late . . ."

"Got any place better to go?"

"Naah."

"Then shuddup. He'll be here."

Out of nowhere a tall, skinny figure materialized. Without preamble, he handed each kid a small glassine bag. "Here's your cut," he said. "Shoot it up or sell it. You know what it's worth on the street. 'S up to you what you do with it . . ."

He turned to go.

"Hey, Bert," spoke one of the kids without a cap. "Thanks. Thanks a lot . . ."

Bert shrugged. "No problem, Al. You earned it. Now, let's get out of here. Couple a cops circulating out there . . ."

The door smashed in. Men with flashlights pounded across the concrete floor. "Freeze . . . we've got you covered. Don't move!"

"It's a bust!" someone shouted. "Run for it!"

Bert grabbed Al's sleeve. "Follow me," he hissed. "Don't make a sound." As noiselessly as he'd come, he melted into the darkness dragging the other boy with him.

"Stop! Stop, or I'll shoot!"

Reflexively, Al paused. Bert didn't hesitate. He jerked Al's arm. "Run!" he hissed.

A shot. Two shots. Al grunted and staggered. Bert tightened his grip and jerked Al into the murky depths of the warehouse.

Behind them they heard scuffling, curses and groans . . . clubs smashing flesh, a body thudding to the floor.

Down the stairs, through a narrow hallway, down a ramp, and out to the dock and the welcome, heavy fog. Al's heart thudded. His breath came in gasps. His shoulder stung like fire. "I've got to stop . . ."

"No you don't. Keep moving. This way . . ."

Bert led, running silently along the splintered dock. Al stumbled along behind him, his heart bursting, head throbbing. Once he fell. Bert turned back, effortlessly hoisted the smaller boy to his feet, and dragged him along.

Not until they were two blocks away did Bert stop. Al was wheezing painfully, gasping for breath. Bert dropped to the ground and Al fell heavily beside him, gripping his shoulder, feeling the warm, sticky fluid on his fingers.

He cried out. "Bert . . . Bert. I'm bleeding . . ."

A match flared. Blood was seeping through Al's fingers, dripping to the worn planks. Al retched convulsively and fainted.

Remembering, Allen Drury shivered. It had been a long road from that abandoned Hunter's Point warehouse — the drug bust, those long weeks of pain and delirium — to Beverly Hills. Somehow Bert had half-dragged and half carried him to a vacant house, made him semi-comfortable and stopped the bleeding. He hadn't known what else to do. Doctors or hospitals would have called the police. He hadn't dared to risk that.

Bert had cared for him like the mother he'd never known. Cleaned his jagged wound with medications stolen from a burgled drug store. Fed him with food smuggled from his home. Finally, still weak and trembly, Bert moved him to a cheap motel, paid for by the sale of his share of the drugs.

The first thing Al knew was waking up in that motel. Outside the familiar roar of commuter traffic told him little. On shaky legs he made his way to the bathroom. And passed out.

Bert found him on the bathroom floor late in the afternoon.

"Al . . . Al, wake up. Wake up."

Al opened his eyes and tried to focus them. A familiar face swam somewhere above him. "Bert . . . is that you?"

"Speak to me, Al. Speak to me! I was afraid you'd never make it. Oh, God . . . you're alive!"

"Alive? Where am I?"

"You're in a motel. I brought you here . . ."

"A motel? But why?"

"You got shot. Remember? That warehouse. The drug bust. We ran. Cops caught the others. They're all in jail. We're the only ones that got away . . ."

"I kinda remember . . . last night . . ."

Bert shook his head. "Not last night . . . two weeks ago. You've been awfully sick. I thought you were going to die . . ."

From that moment Allen Drury pledged his total loyalty to Bertram Collins. They had learned their lesson. No more street drugs. No more gangs. Their own was broken and scattered, most of them serving prison sentences. Somehow they'd both made it to Stanford. There their interests had differed, his to medicine — "I believe I can become rich that way," and Bert's to law — where he sought both wealth and power.

Bert's fierce singlemindedness to his twin goals drove him again and again to the point of exhaustion. But he never gave up. Al's determination couldn't match it. He was more inclined to take it easier, which he did. Too often. He failed first year of med school and had to repeat.

At the end of that first year, Al told Bert, "I can't cut it. Just don't have what it takes."

"That's rubbish, Al. And you know it. I'm going to make it. And *you're* going to make it."

Every step along the way it had been like that: Al struggling. Bert pushing, shoving. Once Al asked, "Why do you do it? You'd be better off without me dragging you down. I'm not as smart as you. Why don't you just leave me behind?"

"No way," Bert said. "We both came from the gutter. From the same ghetto. We've been stepped on, spit on. But, by God, it's not going to sy that way. If there's anything I've learned it's this: It's more important *who* you know than *what* you know. I'm going to learn all the *what* I can, then I'm going to find the *who* to make use of it."

He paced the floor of his cheap apartment. "Al, neither one of us had a chance. But, we're going to make it. *Whatever it takes*, we'll make it. Remember that. Don't ever forget it."

Time came for the finals and Al was sweating blood. This time he *knew* he wouldn't make it. But he gave it his best shot —and passed by a comfortable margin. He was elated.

At Bert's suggestion Al moved to Beverly Hills where Bert had connections. It seemed that Bert had connections *everywhere*. Bert introduced him to an elderly physician who planned to retire in a few years. The chemistry was right between them and Al loved Beverly Hills: the office, the ambience, in fact, everything.

"Thanks, Bert," Al told his friend. "I owe you another one."

Bert grinned. "Sure, sure. One day I'll call the chips in."

For the first time in his life, Al was beginning to feel like somebody. He worked hard under the older man's tutelage, and when the man retired, he offered it to Al for a figure he could handle. Now it was his: a lucrative practice in Beverly Hills. Expensive home and automobiles. On top of the world . . .

And as for Bert. Well, he'd already made a big splash. But now, as legal beagle for Bullion Inc., International, Bert had the world by the tail. The Mercedes handled smoothly. Right on Mulholland, past the University of Judaism . . .

With Bert on his mind, Al dialed a familiar number on his cellular. It was picked up on the first ring. "Bert . . . Al here. Congrats on the new Bullion takeover. You did it again, Bert. You did it again!"

"Thanks, Al . . . and that's just the beginning."

"More to come? What's next?"

"The quacks, Al. We're getting rid of them, driving them out of the country. They're dangerous . . ."

"Dangerous, Bert?"

"You *know* they're dangerous. Drugs is where the money's at, Al. The quacks are telling the people they're better off without drugs. They're telling the people to get off drugs. That kind of nonsense is cutting into our profits . . ." He chuckled coldly and the sound brought chills to Allen's spine.

"That's why we're driving them out of the country. To Mexico. Philippines. South America. The Bahamas. Wherever. We're getting rid of them!"

Drury's mouth was dry. What was he getting himself into? he wondered. Whatever else he was or was not, Drury was neither unforgiving nor remorseless. Even though he differed with his own son on the subject of drug usage, he never intended to drive Jack — or anybody else — out of practice. But, what could he do?

Not knowing what else to say, he mumbled, "Keep me posted, Bert. Okay?"

"Don't worry," Bertram said, "You'll be hearing from me."

Drury was trembling as he replaced the phone and whipped into the circular driveway of his million-dollar home perched high above Sepulveda Pass. Since his divorce, Drury had lived here alone with his son until Jack had gone to med school. He loved this view of San Fernando Valley. Though the sun had set, a golden glow hung over the hills, providing a fitting backdrop for the Valley's glistening lights.

Before climbing tiredly out of the Mercedes, he fumbled for the bottle in his pocket, shook a couple of capsules into his hand and swallowed them without water. He checked the half-empty bottle then slipped it back into his coat pocket.

He had everything a man could desire, but he was miserable. He sighed and set himself for another long, lonely evening.

Collins grinned wolfishly to himself as he unfolded the Fax message and laid it on his desk. He slid a fresh cigar from its wrapper and clamped it into the corner of his mouth. Drury is right, he said to himself. I *have* done it again! He kicked off his Gucci loafers and hoisted his feet to edge of the desk.

He drew deeply at the cigar and eyed the blue cloud with satisfaction. Now the world *is* my oyster, he thought. I've come a long, long way since that day when Phineas Elias tried to ease me out of the picture . . .

Hoping to prevent her marriage to the man, but unable to convince Beatrice that Bertram Collins was not the white knight he appeared, Phineas had the man thoroughly investigated. The result was some very interesting information, including the young man's gang- and drug-related activities prior to Stanford.

The report in hand, Phineas invited the young attorney to his office. Collins chuckled as he remembered the scene. Phineas, proper as ever, simply handed the dossier to Collins and asked, "Do you know anything about this?"

Momentarily thrown off guard, Collins caught his breath, then instantly recovered. Eyes hooded, he took his time leafing through the folder, while his legally-trained brain operated at top efficiency to create a defense. Moments later, he looked up at the old man and smiled guilessly.

"Mr. Elias, I'm going to level with you . . . I *was* born and raised on the wrong side of town. And as a kid I was a gang member for a couple of years . . ."

He adopted what was to become his most convincing manner, one that for years to come would tip the scales in his clients' favor. "But, I realized that route would be a dead end. So, I dropped out of the gang, and turned to education . . ."

He tapped the folder he still held in his hand. "But, in so doing, I made some enemies. Some of them tried to blackmail me into forcing me back into the gang . . ."

Feigning emotion he did not feel, Collins forced his voice to became husky. "But, I never went back. They tried to frame me, to set me up . . . but it didn't work . . ." Dramatically, he placed a hand over his heart. "The charges were never proven. Mr. Elias . . . I am clean."

Phineas reached for the report and Collins surrendered it. "Do you swear that you have never trafficked in drugs?"

"Yes, sir. I swear . . ."

The old man sighed and absentmindedly rubbed the gold handle of his cane. "My daughter loves you . . . and is considering your proposal of marriage . . ."

Collins grinned. "I know, sir . . ."

Phineas arose. When he spoke, his jaw jutted,
his ice-blue eyes were rock hard. Despite himself,
Collins shivered.

"Bertram Collins," Phineas ground out the
words, thumping his cane upon the floor for
emphasis, "I am not finished with my investigation. If
I learn that you have lied to me, you will never
practice law in this city. And my daughter will not be
permitted to marry you. She will be removed from
this country and you will never see her again. Good
day."

As soon as he was out of the old man's
hearing, Collins swore softly. The old fox thinks he
has me. But I outfoxed him! Relentlessly vindictive
and unforgiving, Collins promised himself that the
Phineas Elias influence — either within his home or
without — would never control his life or his destiny.

The Fax message was wrinkled from much
handling. Collins picked it up from his desk and
smoothed it between his fingers. He read it for the
twentieth time. "Congrats, Bert. We did it. Regal and
Custom are in the bag. Just like you promised. That
makes BII Numero Uno in USA! Meet me in Monaco
next week. Bigger bait for higher stakes. Roger K."

"Jane . . ."

A svelte blonde appeared magically. Collins
overtly eyed her expensively-packaged charms. Jane
wiggled herself seductively across the room and
plopped in a chair, exposing a generous area of thigh
in the process. "Yes, Mister Collins . . ."

"Wanna go to Monaco?"

Her blue eyes widened. "Monaco?"

"Yeah, Monaco. Meet her Highness Princess ·
Caroline . . . drop a few megabucks at the tables?
How about it?"

"Well . . . well, yes. But, when? Why . . ."

"When? Friday afternoon. Why?" Bert chuckled.
"To be with me. What else?"

He tossed her a gold plastic card. "Get fixed up for the occasion. Face. Hair. Nails. Clothes. Whatever your pretty heart — and *body* — desires . . ."

"But . . . but, I don't understand . . ."

"What's to understand? The most successful attorney in San Francisco can't travel to Monaco without his secretary, can he?"

As understanding came, a slow blush crept up Jane's throat and face. "Just the two of us?"

Collins nodded lasciviously. "Yeah. Just you and me, Baby. Just you and me."

In Atlantic City, Roger Keller and his chinchilla-clad wife alighted from one of Bullion's stretch limos at Donald Trump's newest, most glittering casino. As the two made their bodyguard-attended grand entrance, Regina asked, "What're we doing here tonight?"

"We're celebrating."

"Celebrating? Celebrating what?"

Unabashedly Roger said, "We're toasting the king — the king of pharmaceuticals — Bullion. And their illustrative chairman of the board . . ." He grinned at her discomfiture.

"But, why?"

"Because I've got my eye on the biggest of them all . . ."

"The biggest?"

"Yes, the biggest. Universe Pharmaceuticals. And then I'll really have the whole world in my hand . . ."

On his veranda, oblivious to the twinkling beauty of San Fernando Valley's nightly light show, Allen Drury sipped his brandy, unaware that Bertram Collins would soon call in the chips owed him . . .

CHAPTER SEVEN

Compared to his father's luxurious suite in Beverly Hills, Jack Drury was quick to admit that his tiny office in East Los Angeles was, to say the least, squalid.

"But now I can have my intellectual freedom," he was telling Carolyn Kemp. "That's something I could never have had when I practiced with my father."

After a quick tour of his facilities, the two were having dinner in Chinatown. She had changed at the office after work and was wearing a light-blue jump suit that complimented both her platinum hair and her aquamarine eyes. Jack still wore the open-at-the-throat shirt and sports jacket he had worn at his office.

"I couldn't help but notice that you and your father had differences of opinion at times," Carolyn said. "But, I thought they were mostly professional dialogue. I never dreamed it would become serious . . ."

"That's what I thought," Jack grinned ruefully. "But then, we've always had our differences. I am of the opinion that all thinking people will differ at least some of the time. But, I never dreamed it would come to this."

He tugged unconsciously at the lobe of his right ear, a habit he frequently indulged in when he was thinking. "Dad's a better than average doc. Good diagnostician. And a good surgeon, probably better than I am. But, then, surgery's never really been my thing. I don't know why. Even in med school it bothered me to slice into someone . . ."

"I never liked surgery either." She looked at her watch. "Well, gotta go. This is my night for swimming . . ."

"And I've got to go back to the office . . ."

He started to get up. "Oh, say, I understand my replacement is a lady doctor . . ."

"Yes. Anne Rush."

"Anne Rush? Shouldn't I know her?"

"Not that I'm aware of. Her father is Bertram Collins. He's an attorney in San Francisco. Her husband's a writer."

Jack was scratching his head as they walked to the parking lot. "Collins. Bertram Collins. Something about the name rings a bell. But I can't quite put it together. Well . . . till next time."

"Thanks for the dinner. Later . . ."

Jack was right, he and his father *had* gotten along well at first. Very well, in fact. Until little things began to creep in. First, it was the noticeable increase of cancer patients they were treating. He spoke of it to his father.

"It troubles me, Dad," Jack said. "It's almost as though it's some kind of an indicator about our practice . . . like we're *attracting* people with cancer . . ."

"Just a sign of the times . . ."

"Perhaps. But it seems to me the same people keep coming back. They never seem to get better. Shouldn't we be helping people to get well, so they don't need us?"

Allen laughed harshly. "Jack, what do you think paid your way to medical school? *Well* people? No, it was sick people. Lots of sick people. Whether they're aware of it or not, a lot of those people just don't want to get well. They need a doctor to help them justify their existence . . ."

That wasn't all that bothered Jack, the other had to do with the drugging of patients, which was such a sensitive issue that he hesitated to bring it up. He was personally very sparing in his administration of drugs, perhaps because of his eclectic reading, which encompassed the total scope of healing literature. While his father was considerably more orthodox in both his reading and his handling of drugs.

Jack finally brought up those personal biases of his. "For one thing, Dad, I'm concerned about the way schools are forcing hyperactive kids to take Ritalin — about a *million* of them this year alone.[6] And our elderly . . . nearly *100,000* died from drugs this year, drug reactions and . . ."[7]

The senior Drury shrugged. "I know, Jack. And that's too bad. But physicians have *always* used drugs . . ."

"I *realize* that, Dad. But not to the same extent that the medical profession does today. I'm concerned about all the new drugs that are coming out all the time . . . and the fact that doctors are prescribing them . . ."

"But those new drugs have been tested," Allen said, his voice rising.

"Not always fully, or adequately . . ."

"What are you getting at, Jack?"

"Well, Dad, for the most part, patients don't realize the danger involved in the use of drugs. Any drugs. All drugs. We do, at least we should. And we should be helping them to get off drugs, instead of writing more and more prescriptions."

Allen shrugged.

"Besides, Dad," Jack pressed, "I'm concerned that we doctors don't tell patients enough about the drugs we give them. Morally, legally, too, we should tell them about the drugs . . . about their limitations. And side effects . . ."

Allen threw up his arms in frustration. "I've tried that, Jack. And patients don't listen. It's almost like they don't want to know. You know that . . ."

Another bone of contention was the regular visits from the drug company salesmen, the detail men. "I think the medical profession's beginning to consider drugs the panacea for everything," Jack said. "And the drug companies promulgate that concept . . ."

Thinking of last night's telephone conversation with Bert Collins, Allen winced. Bullion detail men were the ones who most often frequented his office. But then, he rationalized, those men were just trying to make a living too.

"Perhaps. Maybe yes, maybe no," he countered. "As a whole, we *might* use drugs a little too freely," Allen admitted, "but, you've got to admit, drugs have saved a lot of lives. And I, for one, would hate to try to get along without them . . ."

"I'd like to get along with a lot fewer of them," Jack said seriously. "And, personally, I'm writing fewer prescriptions than I used to."

The older Drury digested that for a moment, before he asked slowly, "Do you *really* think that's wise?"

Jack shrugged. "Basically, yes."

"Just be careful, Jack. Be careful." Brows furrowed, Allen walked away shaking his head.

Allen Drury was out of town for a few days vacation when Reed Janlee breezed into the office. "Hi, Carolyn. You're getting prettier all the time."

"Thanks," she said, a little stiffly, not *too* stiffly, because she knew that Allen liked Reed, and often enjoyed his visits. He smiled pleasantly. "I'll just take that seat over there in the corner. And when you have a moment, will you please tell the high priest that I'm here."

"Sorry, Mr. Janlee, Dr. Drury is gone for the week."

"Well, anybody, then. Who's here?"

"Dr. Jack is here. But he's got a full schedule today," she said, indicating her open appointment book.

"Well, then, since Allen's gone, how about letting Jack know I'm here. I can talk to him. He'll find time to see me."

Carolyn nodded and attached a note to Jack's next patient chart. Though Jack opposed drug use in principle, he liked the chubby, ebullient drug salesman. When he saw the note he stepped into the waiting room.

"Hi, Reed, it will be a while before I can see you."

The salesman waved airily. "No problem. I'll wait." Three hours later, when Jack finished with his last patient, Reed was still there.

"I tell you, Dad, Bullion's got a flock of new drugs. And Reed had a *dozen* of them. None of them generics. All *new*. You know as well as I that it's impossible to create and test that many drugs every year. I think the FDA . . ."

Allen was digging through the boxes of sample drugs Janlee had left. He looked up. "The man was only doing his job. Hmmm, there are a few of these that I'd like to try . . ."

"You can have my share. Excuse me, I've got a patient waiting," he said abruptly as he strode out of his father's office.

The final straw had to do with chiropractors. Jack happened to be reading the account of the court's decision against the American Medical Association in favor of chiropractors when his father walked into his office.

"What're you reading?"

Jack opened the magazine. "Very interesting article about the chiropractor's legal battle against the AMA . . ."

Like most medical men, Allen was familiar with the landmark case. In particular he knew that it dealt with the American Medical Association's refusal to allow chiropractors hospital privileges. Several chiropractors had instituted a class action suit against the AMA, and after eleven years of litigation, the courts had ruled in the chiropractors' favor.[8]

Jack handed the magazine to his father. "Have you read it?"

"No. But, I know about the decision. And quite frankly, I think the judge made a bad call."

"I disagree, Dad, I think this decision will go a long ways toward helping chiropractors and medical doctors to begin working with each other."

"Jack, that's unthinkable!" Allen said heatedly. "It'll never happen. You know that."

"I don't agree. I think the stance the AMA has held against chiropractors was basically wrong. I think it's time the whole matter was settled so we can all get down to the business of getting and keeping people well."

"What do you mean? Work with them. They're not medical men at all. They're bone poppers. Why should they be allowed the use of hospitals?"

"But they are part of the healing tradition, Dad. I know some of those men. Women too. And they know what they're doing. They're helping people get well. People that the medical profession can't do anything for. Face it, Dad, chiropractors can do some things that medical men can't do."

"They can't do anything for patients that I can't do."

Jack spoke softly. "I don't agree. Besides working on the spines and bones of their patients, a lot of chiropractors are nutritionists. And we're not.

We didn't have a dozen hours of nutritional training *between* us in med school."

"They're quacks," Allen retorted angrily. "And whose side are you on? Theirs or ours?"

"I'm not on anybody's side, except the side of fairness. And they're *not* all quacks. You know it. I say, let's work with them instead of against them . . ."

"Why don't you go work with them then?"

"Dad, I'm not a chiropractor. I'm a medical doctor. But I really believe they've got a place in the healing community."

Allen's face was angry red. "You feel strongly about this, don't you, Jack?"

"Very strongly."

"So do I. It's only one of the things we disagree on. In fact, we disagree on about everything."

"That's not really so. We agree on lots of things."

Allen's jaw was clenched. "Look, Jack, don't argue with me. I sent you to med school, and paid most of your bills. And I took you in when you got out. Gave you a place to practice. A place to get started."

"That's right, and I appreciate it."

"I don't think you do appreciate it. It seems to me that you're working against everything I believe in . . ."

"Dad, I'm not against you. It's just that we see some things differently. I'm not *against* you at all."

"Maybe not. But you certainly seem to be against the kind of practice that's supported you in the lifestyle you've enjoyed all your life! And that's all I've got to say about the matter."

Still glaring, the older man turned and stomped down the hall. Suddenly he wheeled and came back. His face was beet red, and he was breathing heavily.

Shaking his finger under Jack's nose, he shouted, "That's not all I've got to say. But this is: unless you can get yourself in line with me, and practice medicine the way I practice it, then there's not enough room for the two of us in this office."

Jack was stunned. "Dad, are you *serious?*"

"I'm very serious. This is *my* practice. I bought it and built it up. I've been treating patients for years . . . the way they want to be treated. And I won't have my way of treating those patients changed. I won't have this practice ruined."

He was panting and sweat ran down his red cheeks. He paused and squared his shoulders. "So, Jack, something's got to give. I can see that you're not about to change your thinking. And I'm not going to change mine!"

The two men stood facing each other tensely.

Jack began, "Dad, I'm sorry. I didn't mean to get you so riled up . . ."

Allen ignored his son's words. "The time has come . . . the time for us to have a parting of the ways. Time for you to move on and start your own practice . . ."

"What?"

"That's right, Jack. I want you to have your things moved out of your office within thirty days."

He stalked out of his son's office and slammed the door behind him. Jack couldn't believe what had just happened. Even less would Jack have believed his eyes had he seen his father at that moment. Seated at his desk, his hands trembling violently, Allen shook a few capsules from the small bottle in his pocket and downed them with a glass of water. He was already ashamed and sorry for the blowup, but too proud to make amends.

That had been six months ago.

When he walked out of his father's Beverly Hills office that day, he'd had no idea what he would be doing next. Carolyn had overheard part of the discussion and stopped Jack in the hallway. "Let's have dinner . . ." she whispered.

Jack looked stunned. "I don't know . . ."

"It's on me. At the Cheesecake Factory. Right after I close the office. Okay?"

He nodded. "I won't be much company. But . . ."

"I insist."

Seated outside in the still-bright sunshine, overlooking the beautiful marina, Jack appeared a little less glum. Carolyn hadn't taken time to change and still wore her white uniform, though she had removed her starched cap.

"I can't believe he did this to you," Carolyn said.

"I can't either. But he did. That's for sure."

"What are you going to do now?"

"That's just it, Carolyn. I don't know. I'm back at square one. Right where I was when I got out of med school: School bills and car payments to pay. Living expenses. But now, I've got no job to pay them with . . ."

To say things had been difficult was an understatement. To be fired from one's own father's office was tantamount to the kiss of death in the closed ranks of the medical profession. Especially in Beverly Hills, from the well-known and respected Allen Drury's office. Not a single door had been opened for him. Jack quite literally had had to start all over again. With practically no resources.

Apparently it had been Jack's defense of chiropractors that incensed his father to the point of dismissing him. Which was ironical, because it was Earl Bailey, D.C., a *chiropractor* that came to his aid, through a brief, three-line ad in the *Pasadena Star News*.

Dr. Anne's Journal

*Wanted, doctor to share office
space / expenses. 794-9988
between 6 - 9 p.m. M-F*

Jack phoned for an appointment, which was
set for the following morning for breakfast at the Salt
Shaker in Pasadena. Jack was ten minutes early. He
recognized Bailey immediately from the man's
description of himself — "About five-eight, 140
pounds. I look like a wrestler. I've got sandy hair. I'll
be wearing a light brown suit."

He waved to Bailey and the man came
bouncing toward his table. That was the term that
came to Jack's mind when he saw Bailey. *Bouncy.*
Like he had rubber springs in his shoes. He wore a
wide grin on a pleasant face, and did, indeed have
the build and look of a wrestler.

He had the grip of a wrestler, too, Jack
discovered when the man shook his hand. "Hi, Earl
Bailey. And you are Jack Drury?"

"Right. Thanks for meeting me so early."

"That's all right. I usually get up early for a
jog and a swim before I go to the office."

As he spoke, he quickly assessed Jack. "You're
a *medical* doctor . . .?"

"Yes. And you?"

"I'm a chiropractor . . . does that matter?"

"Not at all," Jack said, wondering if the words
came out too quickly.

"Good. It matters with a lot of the medical
types." He picked up the menu. "Have you ordered?
No? Well, just go ahead, I already know what I
want."

When Jack had ordered, Bailey said, "Jack, I
want to be as up front as possible. I've never worked
with a medical doctor before. It's an experiment on
my part. But I believe that we — all of the healing
professions — should work more closely than we've
done heretofore."

Jack started to respond, but Earl held up his
hand. "Just let me finish. My office is small. Not
elaborate. Frankly, it's in a semi-depressed area of
East Los Angeles. My clientele are a cross section of
the 'United Nations' types: about every ethnic group
you can name.

"Mostly they don't have a lot of money.
They've got lots of needs. Desperate in some cases.
But they respond to love and understanding. As a
chiropractor I know I can do only so much. So I need
a medical doctor to work with me. I hoped a medical
man would respond. The ad was purposely ambiguous
for that reason."

He paused to take a sip of water. "I figure
that if the chemistry's right we could make a go of it.
And make a worthwhile contribution to our fellow
men.

"Personally, I'm a good chiropractor. Not
brilliant. But good. The deal I'd like to make is this:
share office expenses, including utilities and
receptionist. And speaking of her, the receptionist,
Maria's not a nurse. But she's taking night classes in
a community college . . . medical office management,
or something like that.

"Anyway, we share office expenses, then each
man receives his own fees. How does it sound?"

"Right to the point. Sounds good to me."

Earl smiled easily. "That's how I like to work,
Ben. Now, before I actually interview you, I'd first
like to ask you this question: Do you know anything
about what I call alternative health care?"

"A little, at least by my definition. But I'd be
interested in how you define the term."

"Well, *orthodox* health care, at least as I see it
is . . . No, let me give you the definition used by the
media. Basically, they define the term to mean the
treating a patient with drugs, radiation, or surgery.
Anything other than these modalities, including

chiropractic, nutrition, acupuncture, and so on, they would call *alternative*. Are you with me?"

Jack drew a deep breath. "Earl, frankly, I don't know much about any of these other modalities. Except generally. But I can tell you this, I use as few drugs as possible, avoid surgery when I can, and for the most part, shy away from radiation. Does that answer your questions?"

Bailey grinned and stuck out his hand. Jack grabbed it. And the deal was made.

"Maria, how many patients do you have lined up for me this afternoon?"

Flashing Jack a quick smile, the girl said, "One moment. I will check the appointment book . . ." Using the tip of her pencil, Maria counted aloud, "Let's see . . . the first one is at one-fifteen . . . then two o'clock. And . . . well, altogether you have eight. The last one, a Señor, I mean *Meester* Alvarez, at seven o'clock."

Jack frowned. "*Seven* o'clock. That's a little late, isn't it? I hoped I could leave earlier today."

"I'm sorry, Doctor Jack. He sounded so sick. And *desperate*, I think. He said he cannot get off work any sooner. I think, maybe you take him. No? Maybe I try to reach him. Maybe tell him to come another day?"

"No, Maria. You did right. We're here to treat sick people." He moved to go, then turned back. "Oh, Maria, did this Mr. Alvarez tell you what his problem is?"

"Si, Dr. Jack. He say much pain in stomach. Sometimes he sees blood in his stools. He sound very much afraid." Her brown eyes mirrored her concern. "Not good? Yes?"

Jack smiled at her. "Maria, you're a jewel. You're right. It doesn't sound good. I'm glad you worked him in."

The first two months with Bailey had been
slim pickings and he had barely earned enough to
pay his share of the overhead. If it hadn't been for a
small loan from Carolyn, he couldn't have made it.
She had been very supportive in many ways.

"How about dinner tonight?" She had invited
him on numerous occasions, sometimes at a
restaurant, other times at her condo.

"What are you, prescient or something?" he
asked. "I mean, how did you know that I actually
didn't have two thin dimes to rub together when you
called?"

"A little bird told me."

Jack didn't know till months later that the
little "bird" had been Maria. The evening Carolyn had
"toured" the office, the two had met. The next
morning Carolyn telephoned.

"Maria, this is Carolyn. I met you last night
. . ."

"Oh, yes. You came with Dr. Jack. He like you
a lot."

"He's a very nice man. Anyway, I have a favor
to ask. Can you keep a secret?"

Maria sounded puzzled. "A favor? Secret?
Bueno, I think so."

"Well, I know that Jack, I mean *Dr.* Drury
doesn't have a lot of money right now . . . and, well,
maybe some days he won't have many patients . . ."

"And not make much money, you mean?"

"Yes, Maria. That's right. And when that
happens, maybe you can . . . well, maybe you might
call me. Then I can take him out to eat? Okay?"

"Oh, si, señorita, I mean Miss Carolyn. Yes, I
will call you."

"And, remember, it's our secret. Okay?"

"Si, señorita . . ."

CHAPTER EIGHT

Her grandmother's condition was never far
from Anne's mind and she made it a regular practice
to talk to her every week, and to visit her at least
once a month. Near the end of August, the month she
started working with Allen Drury, Anne made her
plans to fly to San Francisco.

"No, Grandfather," she had said when Phineas
offered to meet her at the airport. "You stay with
grandmother. I'll just take a cab. It's no problem at
all."

Aside from being even tinier and thinner and
more fragile, Magdalene seemed quite her normal
self. As usual, she had dressed herself carefully,
wearing a simple navy dress, trimmed in white,
which fit her to perfection. Her thick, silvery hair
was coiffed in a roll at the back of her head. She
greeted Anne warmly.

"Why, Grandmother, you look wonderful!
You've got the figure of a 16-year old. I'm sure you're
the envy of all your friends."

Magdalene laughed. "You sound just like
Phineas. He treats me like I was a 16-year old . . ."

Phineas chuckled. "Why not? Except for a few
slight changes here and there, you *are* the girl I
married."

The old man, though appearing somewhat
weary from the strain, was dressed as properly as
ever in his ubiquitous three-piece blue serge, with the

heavy gold chain across his vest from which dangled that huge gold nugget Anne had loved to touch as a small child.

"My father found it at Sutter's Fort," he told her once. Today, as usual, Phineas leaned lightly upon the gold-headed cane that was his trademark, without which he was seldom to be seen.

"Keep it up, you two, I love it," Magdalene teased, and Anne was pleased to note that her grandmother's blue eyes had not lost their sparkle. "But, come now, the cook has dinner waiting. And it is special. Everything you like."

All too quickly Sunday afternoon came and Anne prepared to leave. "I insist on driving you to the airport, Anne," Phineas said after lunch.

"Grandfather . . ."

He waved aside her protests, his deep blue eyes twinkling. "Your grandmother has done an excellent job of monopolizing you. Now it's my turn. It will give me a few minutes with you. We can have our little talk in the car."

Magdalene smiled at his subterfuge. "Of course, then you can talk about me . . . and give him the doctor's report."

Anne put her arm around her grandmother's tiny waist. "I have wanted to ask those things, Grandmother. You *look* so well. But I want to know how you are *really* doing . . ."

"Actually, I feel quite well . . . but the tumor is growing. And the doctor says it must come out. Very soon."

"Then what?"

Phineas answered. "He suggests chemotherapy. *And* radiation. I'm against them both. But then, what do I know? What do you think, Anne? You know about these things . . ."

"I'm sorry, Grandfather, but I don't know enough about your situation to give an opinion . . .

but, has he suggested you get another professional
opinion? Or have you considered it?"

The couple looked at each other, and though
no words were spoken, Anne was aware of the
electric communication that passed between them.
She had seen it happen before, and envied them.
They knew each other so well, she thought, they don't
even have to speak. Phineas nodded and turned to
her.

"Anne, we have been thinking about another
opinion. But there's something else. We've been
reading about laetrile . . ." He spoke the word as
though he had spoken it many times before. He
paused and his words hung suspended between them.

"Laetrile?" Anne responded. She had heard
about laetrile, as had every physician. The
controversial drug the quacks used to foster false
hope in desperately ill cancer patients. But what
could she say? Debunk the concept? Bury whatever
illusions — or shreds of hope, however frail — her
grandmother may have entertained?

"Laetrile?" she asked again, grasping for time.

Phineas nodded. "Yes, my dear. Surely you've
heard of it. It's been in all the papers . . . and we've
been wondering . . ."

Anne was aware of the two pairs of eyes fixed
upon her face. She struggled with her integrity. How
could she be true to the pledge she had made at her
graduation, and at the same time be honest with her
beloved grandparents?

I will use my best judgment to help the sick
. . . do no harm. . . . I will not give any fatal drugs
to anyone — even if I am asked. Nor will I suggest
any such thing . . .

But *laetrile*. What did she really know about
laetrile? Only what she had heard, and that from
obviously biased sources. "I will use my *best* judgment
. . ." How can I do that when I know so little? "I will
not give fatal drugs to anyone . . ." But was laetrile

really a drug? Or was it merely a vitamin? A harmless food, a supplement, as some declared?

"I . . . I, really don't know much about . . . about . . . laetrile," she stammered, temporizing.

She saw the puzzled, almost hurt expression in Phineas' eyes. He started to speak, shook his head slightly, and closed his mouth.

"Of course I've heard about laetrile," she went on more firmly. "I've heard that it hasn't been properly tested. And, until it has been, all I can say is, I just don't know . . ."

"I was going to ask you about these things on the way to the airport . . ." Phineas began.

It was Magdalene who rescued them all by injecting softly, "Phineas, my love, I know how concerned you are, but questions such as these put Anne in a rather embarrassing position, don't you think?"

The old gentleman struck his forehead with his hand and spread his arms in a gesture of frustration. "Oi vey! But if we can't turn to our own granddaughter, then to whom can we turn?"

The tiny woman smiled up at her husband who was only a few inches taller than she. "We will call our rabbi . . . and we will talk to our God . . ."

In the end Anne had left them without saying anything more, except to ask for a copy of the doctor's report. When it came, a few days later, she almost wished she hadn't requested it.

". . . the enlarged lymph node was removed . . . sections revealed malignant lymphoma (follicular and diffuse large cell). Other laboratory tests included normal or negative hemoglobin, leukocyte count and differential, platelets, urinalysis (Digoxin (0.9, therapeutic range 0.5-2) . . . Total serum protein was 8.3 (upper limit 7.9) . . . serum calcium was elevated to 11.9. . . .

". . . the patient needs chemotherapy . . . In addition, I suggest 3500 cGy of radiation to the right inguinal area. . . ."

Anne laid the medical report down. "My God!"
"Do you understand it all?" Ben asked.
"Yes, I'm afraid I do. Would to God that I didn't . . ."

The next time Anne saw her grandmother, all of her beautiful silver-white hair was gone and she was wearing a wig. She moved around the house with the assistance of a walker. Her normal weight of 95 pounds had dropped to 85. The lines of pain gave her face a skeletal appearance. But her spirits were high.
"Anne, dear, how nice of you to fly up again."
"I had to, Grandmother. I love you so . . ."
Phineas tried his best to be cheerful, but Anne could detect a gradual wearing down of his strength. He didn't offer to drive Anne to the airport. "I think I'll just stay with Magdalene."
"You should, Grandfather. She needs you . . ."
Nothing more was mentioned about laetrile.

"Is Grandmother in great pain, Grandfather?"
"No, my dear. Not *great* pain. She is uncomfortable much of the time. But the pain isn't so unbearable as it was."
"Please give her my love, Grandfather. I love you both so very, very much."
"And we love you, Anne. I will convey your love to her when she wakes. When are you coming to see us again?"
"I plan to come next weekend."

"Ben, could you come with me next week? You haven't been to San Francisco for a while."

"I was planning to ask you if I could come along with you. So, now that I have your permission . . ." He grinned impishly.

"You have it. So, you'll come?"

"Of course." He became sober. "Anne, if your mother is Jewish, that means that *you* are Jewish. Right?"

"Yes, according to the rabbis, if a mother is Jewish, then the children are Jewish."

"But you don't seem very Jewish."

"Except for the few times when I went to synagogue with my grandparents, I had no Jewish training. My father sent me to Christian boarding schools."

"What does that make you?"

"I don't know. But I believe God hears me when I pray for my grandmother . . ."

"So do I."

San Francisco weather was clear and cold that March. As the airplane made its landing approach, Anne, seated on the right side, caught a breathtaking panoramic view of Alameda, Oakland, the Bay Bridge . . . Treasure Island . . . Alcatraz . . . Angel Island . . . Sausalito and the Golden Gate Bridge.

"I love it. I love San Francisco, Ben."

"Would you like to live here again?"

"Maybe . . . I'm not sure."

Her chemotherapy series behind her, Magdalene's cancer was in remission and she was almost her vivacious self again. Her hair was growing back, but she still wore the wig, and she had gained back some of the weight that she had lost. Nevertheless, a nagging thought kept nudging the back of Anne's mind — was there, *is there* anything that I could do to help her?

Phineas invited Ben to his office Sunday afternoon.

"We have gone over our will," he told Ben, "and I'd like to discuss it with you."

"With me? But I'm not an attorney."

"I know, but it concerns you . . . as well as Anne. Both of you, in fact. Magdalene and I are the last of our clan, the end of the line, so to speak . . . except for Anne."

Ben felt an inner discomfort, a flash of intuition, almost a premonition, and felt somehow saddened at what he was hearing.

"I'd like to read you what my lawyer has drawn up," Phineas said, then thought a moment. "No, you can read it better for yourself." He thrust the three-page document into Ben's hands. Ben read with growing incredulity. When he finished the last page and looked up, about to speak, what he saw caused him to hold his tongue.

Looking very much like the patriarchs must have looked, Phineas sat with his back to the window, framed by a halo of light. His elbows rested on the arms of his chair, his eyes were closed and his hands had formed a steeple. Phineas' lips were moving as though in prayer. The slanting rays of the late afternoon sun turned the old man's hair into pure silver.

An omen, Ben thought, and waited.

"Have you read it?" Phineas asked, opening his eyes.

"Yes, and I must say . . ."

"Please, Ben . . . please. That's the way we want it to be, Magdalene and I. Please allow us to have our way in this . . ."

He smiled and buttoned his coat. "And now, Ben, I believe our cook will be having a fine dinner for us. And we don't want to keep them waiting, do we?"

Ben took the old man's arm. "No, Phineas, we don't."

In the Elias' elegant Nob Hill guest room, long after Ben and Anne had kissed goodnight, Ben stared long into the darkness. He was gripped by a nameless terror that he could not define.

A few weeks later Phineas engaged around the clock nursing care, which Magdalene hated, but reluctantly was forced to accept. "Beatrice comes and talks to me in the night," Magdalene told Phineas. "She was such a wonderful child. She filled our home with joy. She fulfilled the meaning of her name: blessing . . . I miss her. I've always missed her . . ."

"Yes, my dear. I miss her, too."

"If only she hadn't married Bertram Collins . . ."

"But then we wouldn't have our Anne . . . she often reminds me of you when I first met you."

Her smile in the dim light seemed like a halo. "Thank, you, my love . . ."

Phineas turned on his bedside light. "Magdalene, my dear, may I get something for you from the kitchen? A little warm milk, to help you sleep . . .?"

"No thanks. But will you read to me?"

"Of course. What would you like me to read?"

"Perhaps the *Sefer Tehillim*, the Book of Praises . . ."

"Ah, yes, the *Tillim* . . ."

She gave him a beatific smile. "You know my favorite . . ."

"Of course, my dear . . ."

Chapter Eight

And in his melodic chant he began,

> *"O thou that dwellest in*
> *the covert*
> *of the Most High,*
> *And abidest in the shadow of the*
> *Almighty;*
> *I will say of the Lord, who is my*
> *refuge and my fortress,*
> *My God, in whom I will trust,*
> *That He will deliver thee . . ."*

The old woman's lips moved in cadence with his words. Phineas paused and Magdalene's eyes opened wide.

"He *will* deliver me, Phineas . . ."

"Yes, my dear," he said, touching his lips to her hand. She seemed not to notice the tear that dripped upon her cool wrist.

Nights were the worst. She was so uncomfortable, with all those tubes and needles and drains. And the dressing that had to be changed every few hours. The pills and shots for pain.

Shema yisrael, adonai elohainu adonai ehad. Baruch shem kvod malchuto l'olam va-ed. V'a-hafta et adonai elohecha b'chol l'vavcha uv-chol naf-sh'cha m'odecha. . . .

"Phineas . . . Phineas . . .?"

"I am right here, my dear."

"Will you stay with me?"

"Yes. I won't leave you . . ."

"Has the rabbi been here?"

"Yes . . . he will come again soon . . ."

"Did he say the Shema?"

"We said it together."

"Phineas . . . do you see the Shekhinah . . .
the Presence?"

"Yes, my love, it is filling the room . . ."

Magdalene slept hardly at all that night.

Over and over she whispered to herself, "O
thou that dwellest in the covert of the Most High,
And abidest in the shadow of the Almighty, I will
say of the Lord, who is my refuge and my fortress
. . . that He will deliver *me* . . . He *will* deliver me
. . ."

It rained the day of the funeral. Others wore
raincoats and carried umbrellas. Phineas Elias wore
only his usual three-piece suit, the front of it torn
and blowing in the chill wind . . .

Anne had been there with Phineas when her
grandmother breathed her last breath. She had
seldom seen him wear his *tallit*, his Jewish prayer
shawl, but he wore it around his thin shoulders those
last few hours.

And when his beloved wife of over fifty years,
smiled up at him and breathed his name, then closed
her lovely eyes forever, Phineas, with hot tears
sliding down his seamed and weary face, covered his
head with that ancient garment, gripped the front of
his suit coat and ripped it from hem to collar . . .

Intoning as he did so, the traditional blessing
of mourners, *Baruch ata adonai elohainu melelch ha-
olam dayan ha-emet.* "Blessed art Thou, Lord our
God, the true Judge."

Out of respect for her grandfather, Anne bit
her lips until they bled to keep from screaming at
God, whoever and wherever He was. "God, You
promised to deliver Your children. My grandmother
believed You. She believed she would be delivered.
Then . . . *why didn't You deliver her?*"

CHAPTER NINE

"Carolyn, will you please pull the file for . . ." Anne was saying. "Carolyn! What's wrong?"

Seated at her desk, Carolyn had suddenly clapped both hands over her ears and dropped her head on the desk. Her shoulders and back became rigid. A low moan escaped her lips. Outside an emergency vehicle roared past, siren wailing.

Carolyn lifted her head and smiled wanly.

Anne repeated, "Carolyn, what's wrong? Migraine, or . . ."

"Nothing's wrong now." She brushed back her hair with her fingers and straightened her uniform.

"But . . . you . . . I thought . . ."

Carolyn smiled again, as color came back to her cheeks. "It was the siren . . ."

"The siren?" Anne's forehead was furrowed. "Siren?"

"Yes, the one that just went past. Sometimes they catch me unawares, and I just, well, just sort of freak out. I'm better now than I used to be . . ."

Anne pulled up a chair. "Shouldn't we talk about it?"

Carolyn sat down slowly. "I had polio. I was very little. Not quite five at the time . . ."

"That explains your limp."

"Yes, it's much better than when I was younger . . . in fact, I'm not even aware of it most of the time."

"But the siren? What about it?"

"Well, like I said, I wasn't quite five . . ."

Carolyn shuddered. She could never forget the terror of that childhood trauma. Active and athletic, she had been, for all intents and purposes, a very healthy child. The day had been delightfully sunny and warm, she recalled, and she had been playing outside. She became thirsty and ran inside to get a drink of water. It was then, quite suddenly, that the headache began.

"That was the beginning of my nightmare," Carolyn told Anne. "One that just went on and on. They took me to the hospital in an ambulance . . ." She shuddered again. "I still hate them — the ambulances . . . and the awful sirens they have . . ."

"The sirens?"

Carolyn hesitated. "Yes, the sirens. They don't usually catch me off guard like . . . I was so embarrassed . . ."

Anne smiled. "You needn't have been. It's understandable." She frowned in concentration. "Polio? But hadn't you had your immunizations?"

Carolyn nodded. "Yes . . . yes," she said slowly, feeling her way carefully as though through a mine field. Her eyes held Anne's without wavering. "But, you see, I am convinced that the immunization *caused* my polio . . ."

"Caused it?" A look of incredulity crossed Anne's face.

"Yes. Even Dr. Jonas Salk himself — the man who developed polio vaccine — along with other physicians and scientists, believe that polio vaccine can cause polio . . ."[9]

They both fell silent, each engrossed with their own thoughts.

Anne drained her coffee cup and set it down gently. "How long have you been with Allen Drury?"

"Almost ten years. I met Allen, Dr. Drury, through my father. He introduced us about the time I graduated from nurse's training . . ."

"Your father is a specialist . . .?"

"Yes. Oncology. Cancer surgeon. He loves it."

"It's difficult for me to imagine . . . loving oncology. Cancer research, yes. But, treating people with cancer . . ." A shadow of pain crossed Anne's face. "My grandmother . . ."

"Yes, I know. Dr. Drury told me. I'm so sorry." Carolyn reached across the table and touched Anne's hand.

"But, it seems so, so . . . well, hopeless. And there seems to be so little one can do . . . I mean, when she, I mean my grandmother, when she was so sick . . . I felt helpless . . ."

Carolyn nodded. "Yes, I think I understand. We have a number of cancer patients. In fact . . ." she glanced at her watch, "you are scheduled to examine one this afternoon . . ."

"I am? I didn't know."

"Yes. A Mrs. Sorrenson . . ."

"But I don't know any Mrs. Sorrensen."

Carolyn shrugged as she arose. "I don't either. At least I didn't until she called. Anyway, I must get back to my desk." She paused in the doorway. "The woman . . . Mrs. Sorrensen, asked specifically for you. Said she was referred by a friend."

October 18 — Mildred Sorrensen, white female, 82 years of age, came in today. She had been a landscape architect and plant nursery owner/operator for nearly 60 years. Complaining of pain in the stomach. X-ray revealed large mass that looks malignant. Biopsy indicated.
Referred Kemp for second biopsy, second opinion and, if indicated, surgery.

Dr. Anne's Journal

"Ben, the woman's incredible!" Anne was saying. They were enjoying one of Ben's culinary specialties: grilled fish, baked potatoes and tossed salad. She had showered and donned a tailored pink jogging suit to relax in.

She chewed and swallowed a bite of potato. "She's remarkable. Past 80. Eighty-two, in fact. Does all her own housework. And still runs that huge nursery. You know, that one in Malibu, on PCH on the way to our cabin."

Ben nodded and carefully forked a bite of the tender white meat. "She sounds incredible. Must be. To be so active at that age."

"The biopsy showed cancer of the stomach. She goes in for surgery. Tomorrow. Six a.m. . . ."

"What's the prognosis? Good? Fair?"

Anne shook her head. "I don't know. But the woman's attitude is great. She tells me she'll be back to work in a couple of weeks."

"Couple of weeks! She must be fantastic."

"She is."

True to her word, Mildred Sorrensen tapped on Anne's door — and peeked inside — the first day of November. Anne gasped.

"Mildred! You look wonderful! How do you feel?"

The woman was dressed in bright green: green coat and jaunty wool hat, with a bright plaid scarf tossed around her shoulders. "Wonderful. I feel absolutely marvelous. I told you I would."

"Yes . . . but . . ."

Mildred smiled benignly. "But, what? I'm an old woman?" She chuckled at Anne's obvious embarrassment. "Young lady, let me tell you something. Youth isn't everything. It's a lot. But it's *not* everything . . ."

"I know. But, Mildred, I've got to say it. You *are* 82 years old, aren't you? I mean, that's what your records say."

"The number is correct. The adjective is wrong."

"The adjective?"

"Yes, the adjective. It's not 82 years *old*. It's 82 years *young*."

Anne sat down carefully. "Would you mind telling me . . ."

"My secret? I'll be glad to. Doctor . . . may I call you Anne?"

"Please do."

"Anne, the secret is attitude. The mind. Or, better yet, the mind-body connection. Nutrition is important. So is activity. They're both essential. But the attitude is primary . . ."

"I'm not sure I understand."

"Look at it this way. I work with living things. Flowers. Trees. Shrubs. The earth is living. I dig in it. I smell it. Taste it. My life is bound up in life. And in living. Am I making any sense at all?"

"Yes. Yes, please go on."

"It's nearly winter now and many plants are dormant. They seem to hibernate. They go into a state of suspended animation. But they aren't dead. Not at all. They are resting. Resting and becoming rejuvenated. Ebbing and flowing. Ebbing and flowing. Our bodies, our lives are like that. We must learn to ebb and flow as they do — the plants, the living plants. That's why so many plants and trees live such long lives."

She wrapped her scarf around her shoulders. "Cancer. It's an awful word. Plants have cancers too, you know. They get them when they've been hurt . . . or traumatized in some way. Sometimes they overcome the traumas and scars. And live. Sometimes they succumb . . . and die.

Dr. Anne's Journal

"These past two years have been hell for me." Mildred dabbed at her eyes with her handkerchief. "My only daughter was suddenly killed by a drunken driver. My husband died in an airplane crash . . . and I, well I grieved until I got cancer . . ."

She smiled and straightened up. "But I have overcome my scars and traumas. And I'm going to live."

She gathered her things together. "Well, that's enough for today. I must be off." She arose briskly.

Anne stood and walked around her desk. "You will take it easy for a few weeks, won't you, Mrs. Sorrensen? I mean, Mildred?"

The older woman stuck out her hand. "Of course. I'll treat my body properly. After all, it's been good to me for a long, long time . . ." With an airy wave she was out the door.

In the closed room behind her, Anne suddenly felt very old. And very, very tired.

"I tell you, Jack, they're achieving spectacular results down below the Border. Tijuana. And elsewhere. Phenomenal! They're not all quacks like we've heard. Unless you see it with your own eyes it's . . . well . . ."

Earl emphasized his last words with his index finger. "Jack, you've just gotta see it. It's *almost* impossible to believe."

"Tell me about it."

"Well, take that man who came in here a month ago. The one you diagnosed. Colon cancer. Remember him?"

Jack Drury flipped open his appointment book. "Of course. He was in a bad way. Yes, here it is — Roland. Henry Roland, age 55. He's the man who refused surgery. You sent him to American Biologics . . ."

"He came in this morning. Without an appointment. Just wanted to tell us the good news.

106

You were at the hospital, so I saw him. You should have seen him. Full of life. His eyes and skin clear. Full of energy. I tell you, Jack, he's a new man!"

It was nearly eight o'clock and their last patients had gone. Jack Drury and Earl Bailey were seated in their tiny conference room discussing their day.

Jack sipped a glass of Calistoga water, drumming his fingers on the table. "What'd he have to say?"

Earl shrugged out of his white coat and slipped off his shoes. "The man couldn't say enough good things."

"What'd they treat him with? Laetrile?"

Earl nodded. "Laetrile. Megadoses of vitamins. Intravenous and oral. Lots of fresh vegetable juices. Plenty of rest. All of that . . ."

"No drugs?"

"Not according to Roland. Something else, Jack. Every day they herded all the patients together, all of them that could walk — and taught them how to live."

"What do you mean?"

"Just that. Physiology lectures. Nutrition lectures. Dangers of drugs. Pharmacology. The history of medicine. He told me it was like a school room. They used slides, videotapes. Questions and answers . . ."

"And tests?" Jack laughed.

"No tests. But everything else I guess."

"Do they have American doctors down there?"

Earl shrugged. "I don't know. I think so . . . why?"

Jack laced his fingers behind his head and leaned back. "Just curious . . ." He continued thoughtfully. "I'd like to talk to Roland. Then go check out this place for myself. He's the third or fourth patient I've heard about who's taken that

Dr. Anne's Journal

route. And, frankly, it sounds too good to be true . . ."

Earl ripped a sheet of paper from his memo book. "I thought you'd think that. So do I. But I want to withhold my judgment till all the facts are in. So I've got a number for you to call."

"What's that?" Jack said, reaching for it.

"The Cancer Control Society."

Jack's feet hit the floor. He reached for the memo. "Hey, they're only a few minute's drive from here . . ." He was already dialing the number.

CHAPTER TEN

From long experience she knew the signs: tension. Extreme stress. The man, she adjudged to be somewhere in his mid-forties. He was nervous and fidgety, constantly looking at his watch, then checking the time against the waiting room clock. He crossed and uncrossed his legs every few moments. Out of the corner of her eye, Carolyn watched him roll and unroll the magazine so tightly and so often that it had assumed a permanent curled shape.

Phil Crestwood had been thirty minutes early for his appointment. As the hour of 3:00 approached he became even more agitated. He bounced his knees, clenched and unclenched his hands, squirmed in his seat, ran his finger around the inside of his shirt collar. Every few seconds he forcefully cleared his throat . . .

Her intercom buzzed. "Please bring the next patient."

"Yes, Doctor. His name is Phil Crestwood."

She picked up the man's folder and spoke the man's name. He didn't respond the first time. "Mr. Crestwood . . ."

He looked up. "Oh, oh, yes. Yes, Ma'am."

She smiled. "Please follow me."

Neither of them spoke till they reached Examination Room Three. She entered first. "Please remove your clothes and put on this gown," she told him. "Doctor will be with you in a moment."

She turned to go when he spoke. "Do I have a male or female doctor?"

"You asked for a male doctor, so Dr. Drury will be seeing you. Is that all right?"

He smiled nervously. "Yes, Ma'am. Thank you. Just wondered."

As soon as the door closed behind her, Crestwood quickly disrobed and slipped on the hospital gown. Then he hopped up on the examination table and sat there, swinging his legs. A moment later when Drury entered, he looked startled and a wild sort of light came into his eyes. He suddenly began hyperventilating.

"Hello, Mr. Crestwood. My name is Allen Drury."

"Hello, Doctor . . . is this going to hurt me?"

Allen smiled. "I don't think so. Just try to relax and breathe normally. We try to make our patients comfortable."

He sat on a wheeled stool and rolled over close to the examination table, opening the patient folder as he did. Carolyn had taken a preliminary history, and noted his vital signs, which Allen read rapidly, nodding his head, "Uh-huh. Uh-huh."

Then he looked up. "Well, Mr. Crestwood, what can we do for you today?" He smiled pleasantly, a practice that usually helped dispel the patient's fears.

The dammed-up emotions burst in a torrent of run-together words. "I had an x-ray a few days ago and the Red Cross said I should see a doctor because there was a large mass in the left side of my chest!" He gasped for air. "It's getting harder and harder for me to breathe and I can't walk very far without getting l tireout and my heart pounds . . . my mouth is always dry and I don't sleep well and my back aches all the time till I can hardly stand it . . ."

Drury smiled gently and held up his hand. "Hold it. Slow down just a minute. Let me get all of this down." He touched the younger man's knee. "I believe we can help you . . . okay? Now, once again, slower, please tell me what you just said . . ."

Carefully and patiently, Allen Drury listened, touched, probed, examined. Thirty minutes later, he leaned back against the wall. "How long have you been short of breath?"

"I don't know. But it's been getting worse."

"And the pain in your back. How long have you noticed that?"

"About when I noticed being short of breath . . ."

"The same for your chest and shoulder?"

Crestwood nodded. "It's bad, isn't it? I mean, *real* bad?"

Drury smiled encouragingly. "At this point I can't really say. But I suggest we take some x-rays ourselves, along with a few other tests — urinalysis, blood workup, EKG . . ."

"All that? You think it's really bad then?"

Instead of answering directly, Drury asked, "Are you taking any medication now?"

"No. I mean, yes. I mean . . ."

Drury had been writing on the patient's chart. He paused and looked up. "Just think a moment. Are you taking *any* medication. Any drugs, pills or liquid that a doctor prescribed?"

He shook his head. "No, sir."

"Are you taking anything from a drugstore that you got without a prescription?"

"Oh, yes. You see, I watch TV a lot. And I see all these ads . . . for pain, and, and other stuff. So I buy a lot of it . . ."

"And use it?"

"Oh, yes. All of those ads tell us how good doctors say it is. So, I go right out and buy it. Isn't that what we're supposed to do? I mean, I want to take good care of myself, don't I?"

Drury sighed. "Mr. Crestwood, I'm going to have a nurse make a few tests before you go. Okay?

None of them will hurt you at all. Then you go right home and gather up all of that stuff you got from the drugstore and put it in a paper bag and bring it down to my office. Okay?"

"And leave it?"

"Yes, leave it."

"For how long?"

"Until I can see what it is you're taking. Then, I'll write you a prescription for the drugs you need . . . okay?"

Crestwood nodded nervously. "Can I go now?"

"No, you just wait here. The nurse will come right in and make the tests we talked about. Today is Monday. I'd like to have you come back here by Wednesday afternoon. Miss Kemp at the front desk will give you an appointment before you leave. Okay, Mr. Crestwood?"

He arose and extended his hand. "Whatever you do, please *try not to worry*. We're going to do our best to make you feel better. We'll see you in two days. Okay?"

"Yes, sir. I mean, yes, Doctor. I'll be here Wednesday."

Wednesday morning Allen buzzed Carolyn. "Please ask Dr. Rush to come into my office when she arrives. Thanks."

When Anne walked into Allen's office, he was busy examining x-rays. "Good morning, Anne. Take a look at these." He indicated several dark masses on the film.

Anne sucked in her breath. "Whose films are those?"

"Patient by the name of Phil Crestwood." One by one he traced the outlines of the dark spots: skull, chest, shoulders, pelvic area. "Looks bad, doesn't it?"

Anne nodded. "One of the worst I've seen. Apparently spread . . . metastasized, throughout the entire body . . ."

"What would you recommend?"

"A bone scan. There may be more than we see there."

"I agree. I'll have Carolyn make an appointment for him."

Allen and Anne had both gone over the results of the tests and the scan. The blood tests revealed that his alkaline phosphatase levels were sharply elevated and his liver functions were abnormal. Together they placed the bone scan results on the lighted view box and examined them.

Anne caught herself holding her breath.

"It's not good, Anne. Not good at all."

Neither spoke for a while and the room was ominously still. Allen cleared his throat. "What do you think?"

Anne took a deep breath. She felt faint. "Want me to go first?"

"Yes. Please do."

"Well, it looks like he's got either a prostatic or testicular carcinoma . . ."

"I agree. Anything else?"

"Yes, Allen. It looks like the cancer has spread from there to other parts of his body. To some bone tissue . . ." She turned abruptly. "But, isn't that rare? For testicular cancer to spread to the bone?"

"It's rare. But it does happen, Anne. Looks like it has in his case. From the testicles to some ribs, spine . . . yes, shoulder, and . . . possibly even the skull . . ."

Anne sat down suddenly. "Dear God. That poor man. Does he have any idea? At all?"

"I think he suspects it . . ."

Now, sitting next to Crestwood, Allen was having to deal with a very sick patient. The man was frightened. The mere mention of the CAT scan had unsettled him and the procedure itself had greatly unnerved him. Crestwood was doing his best to keep control of himself. He had come directly from work and was dressed in blue jeans and a flannel shirt. He held a baseball hat in his hands, which he was nervously twirling around. To ease the situation, Allen moved out from behind his desk and seated himself opposite the man.

"It's bad, isn't it?" Crestwood burst out.

"Let's just say that it isn't good . . ."

"I'm going to die, aren't I? I knew it all the time!"

"Mr. Crestwood, please calm yourself . . ."

"I knew it . . . I knew it . . ."

"Knew what?"

"You've got bad news and you don't want to tell me."

"Please, Mr. Crestwood. The news isn't good. And . . ."

"I've got cancer, haven't I? Haven't I?"

"Yes, Mr. Crestwood, you do have cancer. But lots of people have cancer and live with it. You could do the same."

The man appeared to shrink before Allen's eyes. He stared at Allen, unseeing, his eyes unfocused. For the first time, his hands were still and he scarcely breathed. Allen leaned toward the man and touched his knee. "Mr. Crestwood, are you all right?"

"Uh . . . uh . . ." He shook himself. "Oh, yes. Yes, I'm okay. It was just a shock to hear for certain that I have cancer." He appeared to calm down and begin to breathe normally. He tried to smile, but the effort stretched his lips so tightly over his teeth that the result was plastic, pasted on.

Allen waited patiently.

Crestwood drew a long shuddering breath. "Well, so I've got cancer. That's what I told my mother . . ."

"Your mother?"

"Yes, I'm not married. I live with my mother."

"Well, Mr. Crestwood, we need to discuss your situation and make some decisions . . ."

"I'm going to have to have surgery?"

"I'm afraid, yes. And the sooner the better."

"How soon? I should tell my boss."

"Today is Friday. You should be admitted Sunday and schedule the surgery for Monday morning quite early. Shall I make the arrangements?"

"Yes. Please do." He snapped his hat on his head and stood up. "Thanks a lot, Doctor." He turned to go.

"Wait a minute, Mr. Crestwood. Don't you want to know where the cancer is located? Who the surgeon will be, and the kind of surgery we'll be doing?"

He shifted his weight from one foot to the other, all the while twirling his baseball hat in his hands. "Uh, no. I don't think I want to know. Just cut it out of me. All of it. Please."

"We'll do our best. And, Mr. Crestwood . . . try to get some rest this weekend. We'll do our best to get it all . . ."

"Thanks, Doctor." Impulsively Crestwood stuck out his hand and gripped Allen's. Then, with a catch in his throat that sounded suspiciously like a sob, he turned and fled.

The microscopic examination of the biopsy, performed while the patient was still in surgery, confirmed the diagnosis of testicular cancer. When the report came, the surgeon nodded and proceeded.

With his scalpel poised, he said to his associates, "We'll be doing a radical left inguinal dissection, remove the left testicle . . . and all of the lymph nodes on the left side of the groin area . . . That's a safety measure, to protect against further spread of the malignancy . . ."

"Will it leave him sexually impotent . . . or sterile?" Anne asked.

"Not actually," Allen said. "But such surgery often leaves the patient *emotionally* impotent . . ."

Just as a hysterectomy often leaves a women, Anne thought, but said aloud, "How tragic."

He nodded. "True. But, under the circumstances he didn't have much choice . . ."

"He actually didn't? None at all?"

Allen looked at Anne sharply. "What do you mean?"

"What would have happened if he'd refused the surgery. Would he have died of testicular cancer?"

Allen shrugged. "Perhaps. Most likely . . ."

"But not certainly?"

"Well . . . no. I don't know for sure."

"How long would he live *without* the surgery?"

"Nobody knows."

"And how long will he live *with* the surgery?"

"Nobody knows for sure . . ."

"Why are you asking?"

Anne regarded Allen soberly. "Just wondering . . ."

December 3 — Phil Crestwood underwent surgery for testicular carcinoma. I asked myself a number of questions regarding his surgery, and other cancer surgery. Does it indeed provide a better quality of life? Quantity? What about Grandmother Elias — did her surgery extend either the quality or quantity of her life? Or was it merely an exercise in futility? As a physician dedicated to the saving of lives, I must find the answers to these questions.

December 5 — Phil Crestwood expired today. Ironically, according to the surgeon, "The surgery was completely successful. But the patient died." The death certificate indicated an embolism that became lodged in the heart. Allen had the task of informing his aged and ailing mother. She was terribly upset. Again, I asked myself, was the surgery necessary? Without surgery he would have undoubtedly lived considerably longer. What would I have done in his position? What would I have done had I been Allen Drury, his physician? Or had I been the surgeon? Questions. Questions.

That night, a Thursday, Ben later recalled, when he ran downstairs to greet Anne, he found her sitting perfectly still in the dead car. She was staring straight ahead, her hands gripping the steering wheel.

When he opened the door, she neither spoke nor acknowledged his presence. She didn't move. A chill of fear raked his spine.

"Anne, dear . . ." he said softly.

She started, her eyes wide and unfocused, seemingly disoriented, as though being suddenly awakened from sleep. "Oh," she said, "Oh . . oh, Ben. Oh, I'm home . . ."

He chose not to alarm her. "Yes, and I have come to personally escort you to your room."

For the first time she smiled. "Ben, that's very nice."

As they negotiated the stairs, he asked, more to make nversation than to seek information, "Busy day?"

"Busy day?" she repeated somewhat distantly. "Oh, oh yes." She shook her head and blinked her eyes.

117

Ben helped her off with her coat. "Actually it's been a terrible day . . ." Suddenly she burst into tears.

"Anne, Anne, what's the matter?"

"I'm just tired. Exhausted. But I'm okay. Just hold me."

He did more than hold her. After she had stopped sobbing convulsively, he lifted her and carried her to their bedroom, helped her undress, and covered her. Moments later when he returned with a cup of hot soup, she was asleep. She looked so weary he didn't awaken her.

It was the sun streaming into their bedroom that awakened her. She was ravenous and ready for the breakfast-in-bed tray Ben had ready for her. "I guess I just conked out last night, didn't I?" She smiled up at him as he arranged the tray and handed her the morning newspaper.

"Sure did. And I had an excellent meal all by myself."

"I'm so sorry, Ben . . ." She patted the bed. "Come and sit down with me while I eat. Oh . . . have you already eaten?"

"Yes, I was up before the sun. And I've already logged a couple of hours on my computer." He regarded her soberly. "You look much better this morning. Feel better?"

"Yes. I guess I was just exhausted."

"You've been working very hard."

She sighed and moved a bite of scrambled eggs around on her plate with her fork. "And I've been seeing an awful lot of terribly sick people . . ."

He grinned. "But what do you expect? You're a doctor."

She nodded. "Yes, I know. But so many of them are . . ." She Shuddered. "They're . . . well, they're *terminally* ill."

She nibbled thoughtfully on the piece of toast. "Ben, I enjoy my work. You know that. At least I enjoy it *some* of the time." She looked up, a look on her face as though appealing for affirmation. "Don't I?"

"I think so. Maybe even most of the time."

"But I'd much rather be in research." Her face was wistful.

Ben's jaw tightened suddenly, reminding her of a bulldog. "And you could be in research now . . . except for your father." His eyes blazed. "I wonder what he's got against research? Or, rather, what he's got against you being in research."

"I'm not really sure. I wish I knew . . ."

"Could it be," Ben went on tightly, "because he's the legal counsel for Bullion Inc.? And he's afraid good research could discourage drug usage?"

"I don't know, Ben." Anne appeared somewhat frightened of his intensity. "Surely, even Father wouldn't be that grasping."

"I'm not so sure, honey. Megabucks can change a man's ethics. And Bullion's certainly got plenty of that . . ."

Anne reached for his hand. "Ben, let's don't get all stirred up over my father. It's a beautiful day, and I'd like very much to drive out to the cabin. Okay? Please."

"But it's only Friday . . . and . . ."

"I was too beat to tell you last night. But I'm going to take today off. I've got to get away from the office. And I feel like I need to go to the cabin for a long, long weekend . . . and, if you could spare the time . . ." She left the rest of the sentence unspoken.

"How can I refuse such an invitation? And it just happens that I can spare the time right now . . ." He frowned slightly. "But, is there something I'm missing? Or overlooked? Something you haven't told me?"

The sudden brightness of her smile was an evasive technique, he thought in retrospect. "Of course not. I just need to get away. And I think you deserve a respite from your work . . . okay?"

His smile was dubious. "That's all? Sure?"

"I'm sure, Ben. Really."

"Well, okay," he said, picking up the tray. "Then, let's go. I can be ready to go in an hour. But you?" he grinned. "How long will it take you?"

She leaped out of bed. "I'll be ready before you are."

He trotted into the kitchen, the magic of her laugh ringing in his ears. Moments later she was singing in the shower.

It was during that weekend at the cabin Ben first realized that something was wrong . . .

CHAPTER ELEVEN

A black cloud engulfs her and she cannot breathe. She opens her mouth to scream, but no sounds come forth. She must run, run, away from the heavy miasma, but her feet seem planted in thick, wet concrete. She twists and turns, but her arms are pinned to her sides. She is sucked into a maelstrom of hopelessness, going down, down, down . . .

The vortex deepens and other helpless creatures sweep past her. She recognizes her grandmother, bound as herself. And her mother . . . her mother, who catches her eye and screams her name. The vortex flattens and fades. Light filters through the slatted blinds . . .

Disoriented, Anne awakens slowly.

Familiarity builds. Those are her books. Her clothes . . .

Abruptly she sits up.

She is in the cabin. Alone. The other side of the bed is empty, the bedclothes crumpled. She shivers and slides down under the covers. There is much to go over in her mind . . .

Memory returns. Anne touches the swollen lymph nodes: under her arms, her neck, her groin. Rubbery and matted beneath the surface. Tender. Painful to the touch. She remembers the elevated blood pressure. Not extremely high, but abnormal. The slow but gradual weight loss . . .

Dr. Anne's Journal

Her skin feels sticky and grimy from the night sweats. She fumbles on her bedside stand for the mirror. Ah, yes, the dark circles beneath her bloodshot eyes.

Has Ben noticed? If so, he hadn't mentioned anything.

Or Carolyn?

"Dr. Rush," she had begun, "you . . . I mean . . .?"

"Yes?"

"Oh, nothing important . . ."

Was it just imagined, or had she caught Carolyn regarding her covertly, eyes narrowed, brow wrinkled questioningly?

She hadn't imagined Allen's awareness. "You're losing a few pounds, aren't you, Anne?"

"Am I?"

"Yes . . . looking good."

"Thanks," she said, but thought, I'm not feeling so good.

"Friday looks rather light, Doctor Rush," Carolyn was saying, "Why don't you take the day off?"

She remembered looking sharply at Carolyn. "Why? What do you mean?"

"Nothing," Carolyn smiled innocently. "You've had a very heavy patient load. Now's the chance to get away. Why not?"

"Thanks, Carolyn. I'll think about it . . ."

By the time five o'clock rolled around she knew Carolyn's suggestion was well taken. She must take some time off . . .

A rap at the door. Ben peeking through the crack. Swinging it wide. "Good morning, Doctor Anne. 'Tis a lovely day. And how is m'lady this morning?" He swept into the room, bringing with him a fresh breath of the whole out of doors.

"Better. Much better." She stretched luxuriously. "But I just might stay in bed for a while."

"Breakfast? Now? Or later?"

She slid down deeper. "Later, I think. Okay?"

He kissed her lightly on the top of her head. "Anytime. I'm going out to chop some wood. I'll peek in after a while. Love you."

"Love you." She closed her eyes. She heard him standing there, felt his eyes upon her. What was he *really* thinking? Then she heard him tiptoe out and softly close the door, leaving her alone again with her fears.

"What do you mean by IIMP?" Jack asked.

"IIMP. That's the acronym we coined to spell out what we call Individualized, Integrated Metabolic Programs. It defines our total metabolic/nutritional approach to patient treatment."

Jack Drury was seated in Michael Culbert's office in Chula Vista, California. Culbert is the Director of Public Relations for American Biologics-Mexico, S.A.[10]

"And just what is that individualized, integrated metabolic program? Sounds like something I should know about."

"We think so," Mike said easily. "We think it's the 'cancer answer,' to use a pun . . ."

"Laetrile?" Jack asked bluntly. "Isn't your IIMP just another way of saying laetrile. Just an umbrella term you use to catch people off guard?"

Mike chuckled pleasantly. "No. Not really. It includes laetrile, of course. But in and of itself IIMP isn't laetrile."

"Then what is it?" Jack asked. "Look, I don't want to appear obnoxiously pushy or aggressive, but I've got to know. I've got some pretty sick patients in LA, and I don't have a great deal to offer them . . ."

"Except the usual surgery, radiation and chemo?"

"That's right. And a little nutrition thrown in. But, frankly, Mike, my partner and I, we're just stumbling around in the dark."

Mike steepled his fingers in a characteristic gesture. "I know what you're talking about, Doctor . . ."

"Please call me Jack. Okay?"

"Okay. But, Jack, I've heard that story hundreds of times from doctors like yourself. And I, that is, we, want to help you. All of you, doctors and patients alike."

"You do?"

"Yes, we don't have any patent on what we do. Our doors are open to everybody. Our therapies are an open book. We'll tell you what we do. We'll share our case histories with you . . ."

Jack drew in a deep breath. "You know what they call you up in LA . . . everywhere, I guess."

"Of course I know. We're the 'cancer quacks.' We're the ones who feed people a few apricot pits, take their money, and don't do much else. Right?"

Jack nodded. "I guess you've heard it all . . ." He thought a moment. "But why here? South of the Border? Why don't you do what you do in the States?"

Mike looked stern for the first time. "Jack, you of all people should know the answer to that. American doctors get thrown into jail for treating people with the modalities we use. You know that. And if you can't think of some doctors who've had their licenses revoked, I'll name a few of them. I've got a whole file drawer about them."

"But, why, Mike? Why?"

"I'll tell you why. It's basically a matter of economics. We help return people to wellness down here. We don't drug, cut and burn them to death. We don't treat them like statistics. We treat them like whole people. We individually analyze each patient, determine his problem. Then design an IIMP — there's that name again — we design an individualized, *integrated* metabolic program for that patient, and for that patient alone."

"For a lot of money?" It was a question, not a charge.

Mike raised his eyebrows. "A lot of money?" He chuckled. "I guess that's a relative term. A patient can spend a month down here, receive all the tests, all the therapies, including room and board and whatever supplements or medications he needs . . . for how much?"

Jack shook his head. "I don't know. You tell me."

"That whole month down here — on the average — will cost a patient *less than a single week* in an American hospital. And that includes *everything* we do for them!"

"But will that cure him, or her, of cancer?"

"Cure, my friend, is a word we don't use down here. We have never *cured* anybody of anything. Nor do we pretend to do so. But our record — in terms of people returned to wellness — speaks for itself. It's a great deal more impressive than the record the American Cancer Institute can boast of."

"But, if you don't cure people of cancer, what do you do?"

"We *detoxify* people. We rid them of the accumulated poisons that have made them sick. We teach them why they got sick in the first place, and how to live so as not to get sick. We feed them good food and teach them how to do the same for themselves . . ."

"Is that all you do?"

"Not by a long shot, Jack. American Biologics, AB-Mexico, offers the patient the world's first total assembly of *all* major metabolic/nutritional and eclectic modalities. The latest in advanced and innovative diagnostic and monitoring techniques.

"And, at the same time, while availing itself of the most sophisticated standard therapies and testing, diagnostic and analytical equipment . . ."

"Whew!" Jack said. "And . . ."

Mike waved him down. "That's not all. AB-Mexico's got a fully licensed and accredited international on-site staff, backed by consultants from around the world and a complete backup team of physicians and nurses . . ."

He paused to take a breath. "We're very proud of what we are. Because we're a full-service complex with both out-patient and hospital facilities. Around the clock. Along with a restaurant and laboraty . . ."

Mike grinned. "That's not all. But that's a starter."

Jack looked down at his hands. "Almost every day I hear of some more sick people coming down here. And I wondered why."

"I hear that all the time. Now I know why they come. You see, Jack, you doctors north of the border aren't doing a very good job of helping people to get well. And to stay well. Because, if you were, we'd be out of a job."

He chuckled. "I keep telling doctors how they can keep people from coming to us . . ."

"How?"

"By getting people well. If you did that, then people wouldn't be flocking to us by the thousands. All you orthodox doctors have to do to put us out of business is to start doing a good job with cancer . . ."

Jack arose and stuck out his hand. "Thanks, Mike." Then he spoke slowly and thoughtfully. "I'm not so sure that I'd call myself an *orthodox* doctor anymore. If I ever was one . . ."

"Meet me for lunch?" Jack asked.

"Anytime on *any* Friday," Carolyn answered. "I'll be glad to get away from here for a couple of hours."

"How are things at the Drury Clinic?" Jack asked her when they met at The Greenery.

"About the same, I guess. Busy. Busy. Sick people . . ."

"Take a look at this."

"What's that?"

"It's a brochure I just picked up in Chula Vista . . ."

"American Biologics?" Carolyn accepted the brochure. She looked at Jack with surprise written across her face. "You've been to one of those quack cancer clinics?"

Jack grinned. "Read it. Then ask me about it. You might begin using another descriptive term."

"But, Tijuana?"

"That's right. I just came from there a couple of days ago."

"And . . .?"

How lovely she looks, Jack thought, and realized how little there was to his life besides work. Aloud he said, " Just read it, Carolyn. Read it. Then ask me what I think . . ."

Driving back to the Drury Clinic Carolyn wondered if Jack ever thought of her as a woman instead of just a nurse. She laid her purse and brochure on her desk and promptly forgot about it.

The general offices of Bullion Inc., International, towered high above Central Park, with the office suites of the president and chairman of the board occupying the entire 65th floor. Roger Keller slammed down the receiver and buzzed his secretary.

"Get Bert Collins on the line."

"Yes, Mr. Keller."

Angrily chomping his unlit cigar, Keller paced around the spacious room like a caged tiger, ignoring the glorious view of the city. When Collins came on the line, without preamble, he demanded, "Do you know anything about laetrile?"

"Sure do, Roger. What do you want to know?"

Without answering, Keller demanded again, "Know anything about those south of the border cancer quacks?"

"Quite a bit. There's a bunch of them. Any in particular?"

"Yes. Get in touch with Drury. Jack Drury, Allen's son, is getting too friendly with one of them to suit me. Allen will tell you which one it is. I want him to stay away from those cancer clinics. Starting now. Now. Before he gets any deeper . . ."

"Any suggestions?"

"Just use your head. Don't involve Bullion. Understand?"

"I understand."

With a final click, the conversation was finished.

Allen Drury was headed home on the 405 when his car phone buzzed. "Yes?"

"Allen, this is Bert."

"Yeah. Hi. What's up?"

"You owe me one. Remember?"

"Sure. What can I do?"

"I understand Jack's getting involved in one of those south of the border cancer quack outfits."

"He is? What do you mean?"

Bert's voice switched to his witness stand tone. He purred deceptively. "I think you know. Anyway, find out. And stop him."

"Stop him? He's his own man, Bert. He's not a kid anymore. How can I stop him from doing anything?"

Chapter Eleven

"That's your problem. I'll check back." He hung up, leaving Allen literally holding the phone.

CHAPTER TWELVE

Earl Bailey tossed the brochure on his desk. He looked up. "It's impressive . . . but does it mean anything?"

"I think so," Jack Drury said. "Let's put it stronger. I *believe* they are legit. But they're not the only ones in Mexico. Or the world, for that matter. Since I talked with the people at American Biologics, I've learned of at least a dozen cancer clinics in Tijuana, Mexico City, West Germany, the Philippines, Greece . . . all over the world . . ."[11]

"Except for the United States."

Jack nodded. "Except for the United States."

"And the reasons are obvious." Bailey was not asking a question.

"Obvious as little green apples. Megabucks. *Billions*, no *trillions* of dollars. And who is making all of that money? The medical/pharmaceutical monopolies. Or cartel. Or, if you please, the supermeds. Or the medical industrial complex. That's who."

"What are we going to do about it?" Bailey asked.

"Well, partner, mightier forces than ours have come up against them . . . and have bit the dust. Been put out of business. And I don't intend to join the ranks of the losers."

"Then, what're you going to do?"

Jack adopted a karate stance. "I don't intend to come against the supermed/pharmaceutical cartel head to head . . ."

Bailey raised his eyebrows. "Oh? Then what . . .?"

"I'm going to enlist . . . in the growing ranks of the pro-choicers . . ."[12]

"What do you mean by that?"

"I don't know for certain . . ." Jack began to pace. "But I can tell you this: I'm tired of seeing my patients get sick and die. Without hope. I want to give them hope . . . and something besides hope. I want to give them their lives.

"I want them to have choices . . . choices about the kind of medical treatment they want. And I'm going to do everything I can do to see that they get it . . ."

He stopped pacing and stood toe to toe with Bailey. "I'm not trying to put the drug industry out of business . . . sometimes drugs are necessary. And I'm certainly not trying to put the surgeons out of business. Sometimes surgery is needed. All I want to do is eliminate the monopolies that control a patient's choice. And to give him freedom . . . freedom for him to choose what's right for himself . . ."

Bailey jumped to his feet and applauded. "Bravo, Jack!" he said. "Got room for some help in your campaign?"

Jack Drury grinned. "Shake, pard. . . if you want in, you're in. I don't know what this'll lead to, but I surely like my patients to get well. Even if the sick ones do pay the bills."

Maria was smiling at one of Earl Bailey's antics when the phone buzzed. "Good morning. Medical Clinic," she answered pleasantly.

A harsh voice ground out. "Tell Jack Drury to call his father!"

"Excuse me," Maria said, "may I have your name, please?"

The line went dead.

She hung up slowly. Bailey noted the puzzled look in her eye. "What was that all about?"

"I don't know. It was a man. A voice I didn't recognize."

"But what did he say?"

"He just said, 'Tell Jack Drury to call his father.'"

"That's all?"

She nodded. "That's all. No, 'please,' 'thank you' . . . or anything." She scribbled a note and started to rise. Bailey took it from her hand. "I'll give it to him, Maria. I wanted to talk to him anyway."

"What?" Jack said. "He told Maria what?"

"She didn't recognize his voice and he refused to identify himself. All he said was, 'Tell Jack Drury to call his father.'"

Jack took a deep breath. "He's angry about something. I'll give him a call . . ." He reached for the telephone.

Carolyn took the call. "Hi, Carolyn . . . Jack."

She covered her mouth and spoke directly into the phone. "Hi, Jack. Nice to hear your voice. What can I do for you?"

"Well, I think Dad wants to talk to me . . ."

"Okay, I'll buzz him."

When she connected them, Jack said, "Hi, Dad. I got a message that you want to speak to me."

"Just a moment." Allen got up and closed the door. "Yes, Jack, I do. I just got word that you've been hanging around with some of those quack cancer clinics . . ."

"Well, I've visited one of them, if that's what you mean." Jack was puzzled. "It was a nice place. Clean and . . ."

"Leave it alone, Jack." Allen growled.

"What?" He was startled by the anger in his father's voice. "What did you say?"

"They're dynamite, Jack. Back off and don't mess with them."

"I don't understand. They seem to be doing a good job . . ."

A note of anxiety crept into Allen's voice. "Jack, for God's sake! For your own good . . . and for mine, leave them alone."

"Dad," Jack said softly, "is there something wrong? Is there some *reason* why I shouldn't deal with those clinics?"

Allen was aware that his hand on the telephone was slippery with sweat. Despite himself, his voice shrilled. "Yes, there is. But, I . . . I can't, I mean . . . just don't go back there."

"Dad, Dad . . . what's wrong?"

Unable to control himself any longer, Allen took a deep breath and gently lowered the phone in its cradle.

Jack held the silent phone in his hand for a long moment. Shaking his head in puzzlement, he hung up.

That evening Jack's telephone was ringing as he ran up the stairs to his apartment. He grabbed it. "Hello . . . Oh, hi, Carolyn. What's up?"

"That's what I'd like to know?"

"What do you mean?"

"What did you say to your father that shook him up so?"

"Shook him up?" he answered cautiously. "Like what?"

"He was upset and depressed all afternoon. What did the two of you talk about?"

"Well," Jack began, "it was a mighty curious conversation. I'm not really sure what it was all about . . ."

"Oh? What do you mean?"

"Well, he warned me to keep away from what he called 'those quack cancer clinics.' And when I asked him what he meant, he, well . . . he sort of went to pieces. Then hung up."

"That's strange. And you don't know why?"

"No. I haven't got the slightest. That's really the weird part of it. He was saying something about it being for *my good* as well as for *his good*. When I asked him what he meant, he started talking funny, like he was all stressed out. Then he told me he couldn't tell me any more than that . . ."

"I don't understand it, Jack."

"Neither do I. Was there anybody else in his office?"

"No. Not then. He hasn't seen anybody today except patients."

"Strange phone calls?"

She thought a moment. "No, none that I can recall. Why? Do you have something in mind?"

"No, Carolyn, I don't. Just trying to put it all together."

Light filtered softly through the drawn drapes when Anne opened her eyes. Momentarily she couldn't remember where she was. Awareness dawned and she stretched. The sudden stab of pain in her axillary and inguinal nodes took her breath. She gasped, and it all came rushing back.

"Dear God, don't let it be . . . oh, God . . ."

She was sobbing when Ben quietly opened the door. He dropped to his knees beside the bed and gently took her into his arms. Without a word, he ran his fingers through her hair and kissed her cheek. After a while she relaxed in his arms . . .

Alex Cranston completed his examination. "Anne, I won't try to dissemble with you. That's not my way. Besides, it wouldn't work. You know too much."

Anne nodded, unsmiling.

"First, a question . . ." His grey eyes, not unkind, but professional, caught and held hers. Her eyes didn't waver.

"Yes . . ." Her voice was low with fear and tension.

"How long have your nodes been swollen?"

Her eyes wavered. "A couple of years . . ." she whispered.

"A couple of *years?*" Cranston echoed in unbelief.

"Yes . . . at first I thought . . ."

"That it would go away?" Cranston completed the sentence. "I don't understand. You of all people. A physician."

She drew a long, shuddering breath. "I guess you don't . . . actually, can't understand . . ." Her eyes begged mutely for his support.

"I'll try to understand." He smiled gently.

"There's hardly been a time in my growing up years . . . since I became a teenager, I guess . . . when my lymph nodes weren't painful. At least part of the time."

"And you never told . . . *anyone?*"

She shook her head. "No . . . I couldn't."

"But, why?"

"I was afraid . . . I guess I was always afraid . . ."

"Afraid of what?" Cranston asked.

"Everything. My father most of all. You see, my mother died when I was born. And he, well, he raised me. Or, *had me raised.* I seldom ever saw him. He was always gruff and angry. Angry at me, I thought. And I tried . . . I tried so desperately to please him . . ." She was crying, but unaware of the hot tears that dripped from her chin.

"I guess it was when I was a teenager, in high school . . . when I first noticed my lymph nodes were swollen . . ." She shivered, remembering.

"So, I . . . found a copy of the *Merck Manual* in daddy's office. He does a lot of legal work for doctors. And I read about it . . ."

She tried to smile, but failed. "It wasn't very reassuring. So I just kept it to myself. Never told anyone. Ever."

Cranston was shaking his head in disbelief. "You poor girl. You must have been terrified."

"I was," Anne said, now in control of herself. "Most of the time. Then I met Ben. And he was the most wonderful thing . . . person, in my whole life. But I was afraid that if I told him I was, was . . . sick . . ."

"But, Anne, most of the time you *weren't* sick. It was just that you were . . ."

"I know that now, Doctor. But by the time I learned that, I, I just . . . accepted it as part of life . . ."

Cranston cleared his throat. "Well, Anne, it's time to do something about that condition . . ."

"A biopsy?" she said. It wasn't really a question.

"Yes. The sooner the better. I strongly suggest that you come in tomorrow . . ."

Anne drew a long, shuddering breath. "Okay," she whispered. Her legs felt rubbery when she arose to go. Cranston gripped her elbow and walked her to the elevator.

She didn't go directly home. Instead, she drove to Ocean Boulevard and parked. As she so often had done when troubled, she seated herself on a bench overlooking the Pacific and fed the horde of pigeons that seemed to know her. Somehow the birds and the incoming tide served to calm her weary, fearful spirit.

In his Mulholland mansion high above the San Fernando Valley, Allen Drury finished his brandy and set the glass down carefully. Fear moved in him like a live thing. From long, firsthand experience, he knew Collins' methods and knew the man expected results. Demanded them in fact.

Once again he dialed his son's number. And again he got the answering device. "Hello, this is Dr. Jack Drury. Please wait for the beep . . ."

Allen angrily slammed down the telephone. "Damn, Jack! Why doesn't he come home? I've *got to* talk to him again." For the thousandth time he wished he hadn't fired Jack and that the two of them could work together as a team . . .

In the darkness of their Santa Monica condo, Anne clung to Ben. She feared the long night. And the morning that would follow. She tried, but could not force herself to tell Ben about the biopsy . . .

CHAPTER THIRTEEN

Even before she became ill, Anne's emotions were mercurial, and her mood swings often difficult for her to handle. But since receiving the positive biopsy report from Dr. Cranston's — which she still had not mentioned to Ben — she feared to allow him out of her sight.

Ben tried to accommodate her. But, despite her fears, it became imperative for him fly to New York and spend the day with his publisher and make publicity plans for his new book.

"It'll be a turn around trip," he said. "I'll leave early. The publisher will meet me at Kennedy for a couple of hours, then I'll get on the airplane and return. Be home tonight . . ."

She clung to him, finally releasing him. "Well, okay." She smiled wanly. "I'll miss you all day."

"I'll miss you, too. But I'll hurry home."

Not content with waiting at curbside, as Ben had suggested, Anne insisted meeting him at the gate. The moment he spotted her, Ben knew something was wrong.

He guided her toward the escalator. "You've been crying Anne. Something is wrong. What is it?"

"It's grandfather . . . he . . . he died today."

Ben stopped so suddenly that passengers bumped into him. He moved aside to let them by. "Grandfather Phineas *died?*"

"Killed. Killed by a hit and run driver . . ."

"I can't believe it. I talked to him on the phone just this morning. We were talking about . . . oh, that doesn't matter. What happened?"

"It was five o'clock. Grandfather had just left his office. He doesn't have to, but he still goes there every day . . ."

"Like he's done for the past fifty years or so," Ben interjected.

"Yes. Such a dear, dear, wonderful man. He was waiting at the corner for the light to change. The driver cut the corner sharp and struck him. Grandfather never . . . he never knew what hit him . . ."

> *April 20 — Grandfather Elias was killed today by a hit-and-run driver. I can't bear to think of him as being gone. He loved me. Now his love is gone. And part of my life went with him. I don't want him to be gone. I miss him terribly already. Grandmother was sick for so long, and suffered so much. That was terrible. But, maybe not as terrible as losing Grandfather all at once. With no warning.*

Again it rained the afternoon of the funeral. Feeling cold and forlorn, Anne snuggled into Ben's arms. Driving back to Nob Hill, the dark, wet trees that slipped past the limousine seemed to scratch dark, wet furrows on her soul.

She shuddered. "Don't you leave me like they did, Ben. Please." A tight sob escaped her cyanotic lips.

He tightened his grip upon her. "I won't, my darling. We'll have many, many years together. I promise . . ."

She sat up suddenly and gazed intently into his eyes. "Will we, Ben? Will we have *many* years together?"

He kissed her gently. "Yes. Many years."

April 22 — The two most beloved people I have ever known have been wrenched from me. Along with their love. What would I do without Ben and his love? The ominous dread I have battled for so many weeks is upon me in full force. My grandparents' deaths: are they omens of some kind? The deep pain I feel at their loss is almost more than I can bear.

The day after the funeral Anne called Bertram's office. "Hi, Daddy. It's Anne. May I come and see you . . .?" she began.

"Where are you?" he demanded.

"At Nob Hill. Ben and I will be here for a few days . . ."

"What do you want?" he asked cautiously.

"I've just got to talk with you. That's all . . ."

"Make it around four-thirty this afternoon."

"Yes, Daddy . . ."

"Don't be late. See you then." He broke the connection abruptly.

She dressed carefully for the meeting. "How do I look?" she asked Ben. He whistled. "Like a seventeen-year-old getting ready for a date. Smashing!"

Ben drove her and promised to meet her in Collins' foyer half an hour later. She felt less than enthusiastic about the meeting. The very young, stylishly-dressed secretary was new and didn't recognize her.

Anne tried to quell the butterflies in her stomach and appear calm as she leafed through the expensive selection of magazines in the ultra modern law office waiting room.

It was nearly a quarter till five before the receptionist said, "Mrs. Rush . . . pardon me, *Dr.* Rush . . . Mr. Collins will see you now . . ." and directed Anne to her father's inner sanctum. Collins did not arise or move from behind his massive desk when Anne entered the room, but simply motioned her to a chair. She was subliminally aware of the psychological power that huge desk provided him.

Nevertheless, despite that awareness and her planned resolve, Anne realized that she *was* intimidated. Suddenly she felt like a little girl again in her father's presence, and found herself twisting her handkerchief between her fingers.

Collins looked up from a paper he'd been reading when she entered. "Well, Anne, you said on the phone that you wanted to talk to me . . . what is it?"

She cleared her throat and came directly to the point. "Did you know that Grandfather died . . . I mean, was killed a few days ago? The funeral was yesterday . . ."

"Yes. Yes, I know. I was in Switzerland on business. Just got in late last night." He laid down his pen. "You said there were a couple of things . . ."

She hesitated. Just how much should she tell him? All of it, she decided suddenly. "Daddy, I believe I have cancer. The same kind that Grandmother had . . ."

"You *believe* you've got cancer?"

"Yes. I had a biopsy a few days ago. I don't have the report yet. But . . . well, I know the signs . . ."

If the news disturbed Collins, he didn't show it. He did have the graciousness to offer, "I'm terribly sorry, Anne. I expect, ah, that you'll be having surgery . . .?"

"I'm not sure yet. That is, I haven't decided
. . ."

For the first time Collins showed emotion. "For
God's sake, girl, what do you mean, you haven't
decided?"

"I'm thinking . . . at least I'm considering
going the laetrile route . . ."

Her father's immediate reaction startled her.
He shoved back his chair and leaped to his feet.
"Laetrile!" he shouted, in the loud voice that had so
terrified her as a child. "Laetrile? In heaven's name,
what for? That stuff's nothing but a ripoff!"

"But Daddy . . ." she attempted.

He refused to be silenced. His tirade against
laetrile and the "Mexican cancer merchants" unnerved
her. His harsh words engulfed her, overwhelmed her.
Frightened her. But, even worse, evinced no shred of
concern for her well being. Instead, he seemed to be
waging a verbal vendetta against alternative
medicine, which served only to further confuse her.

Finally, she did as she had so often done as a
child. She slunk out of his office — shaken and
unsure of herself. She was very quiet that evening.
Ben did not press for details.

Ben and Anne remained at Nob Hill, almost
an institution itself, for several days, settling estate
matters. They decided to keep the housekeeper, maids
and grounds keepers on and the house open
indefinitely, to the immense relief and gratitude of
the staff. Though they made no immediate decision,
they discussed the idea of relocating in San Francisco.

"I could write as well here as I could in Santa
Monica," Ben said.

"But I don't want to leave our Malibu cabin
. . ."

"I know," he agreed. "The isolation, the quiet
of the cabin is like balm to our souls."

Dr. Anne's Journal

"And I so need that balm, Ben. So very much . . ."

A week after the funeral they took the 8:00 a.m. American Airlines flight to Los Angeles. As the airplane lifted from San Francisco International Airport and gained elevation above the Bay, bright rays of the sun caressed the towers of the Golden Gate Bridge.

Like a bright omen, Ben mused. Perhaps our circumstances will now improve . . .

Still despondent from the deep void in her life — her grandfather's death and her father's lack of either concern or understanding — Anne was saddened by the sight. *Perhaps the Gate is closing upon me,* she mused, *and this is our farewell.*

Anne closed her eyes and tried to sleep. Beside her Ben, noting the deep stress lines in her face, longed to wipe them away. If only she didn't feel so deeply about her patients. He promised himself that he would watch her more carefully and try and help her to conserve her energies . . .

Feigning sleep, Anne wondered, wondered, *Is it foreordained that I must die the way my grandmother died?*

She had difficulty resting that night, but shortly after dawn had fallen into a deep sleep. Ben carefully eased out of bed and showered. They had decided to spend a long weekend at their Malibu cabin, and after nearly two weeks away from it, Ben was eager to get back to his computer. He had just poured himself a cup of coffee in the kitchen when he heard her scream . . .

"Ben . . . Ben! Where are you, Ben?"

She was sitting upright in bed, a look of terror upon her face when he entered their bedroom and knelt beside her. "Anne, Anne, what's wrong?"

She moved into his arms. "Oh, Ben. It's you. I thought you were . . . were . . ."

He kissed her wet cheeks. "I was what? Had gone?"

She tried to speak. "Yes. No . . . oh, Ben. I dreamed you had died . . . I awoke and you were gone . . . and I couldn't stand it . . . to have you gone . . ."

She clutched at him with her hands. He cradled her tightly against his chest while painful sobs convulsed her. Finally the sobs and shudders ceased. He gazed down into her red, swollen eyes. And bent and kissed her long lashes.

"Ben . . . Ben, please promise me . . . will you promise?"

"Promise you, Anne? Promise you what?"

"That you won't let me die alone."

"I promise," he said. And a cold chill slid down his spine. Dear God, what is she talking about?

She sought and tightly gripped his hands with strength he didn't know she possessed. "Oh, Ben, I need you so very much."

She made love with him fiercely, demandingly, clutching at him as though she could not get enough of him. Then, exhausted, she curled up in his arms, trembling like a frightened child. He held her tightly until he felt her tense muscles gradually release and her breathing become regular.

How pale she looked. And thin. Unarticulated fear clawed at his vitals. Reluctant to leave her again, Ben leaned on one elbow beside her and watched her while she slept.

> *April 30 — The heaviness seems never to leave me now. At the office I am faced with depression, disease and death. The ghosts of my beloved grandparents talk to me day and night. My father's harsh anger directed against doctors who practice alternative medicine. I don't understand. It must be connected some*

145

*way with his business. Nothing else
seems to move him. Oh, God, what shall
I do? The pain is becoming more
intense. More frequent. Ben must be told.
But, how? What can I tell him? Was it
Job who declared, "What I feared has
come upon me; what I dreaded has
happened to me"? I am so wretched and
so afraid.*

They had designed their cabin with huge
windows on every side so as to take advantage of
their magnificent hilltop view. From their kitchen and
breakfast room they could catch the morning sun.
While the living room and master bedroom both
overlooked an unparalleled panoramic view of the
vast Pacific coastline.

Propped up in bed with her hair fanned
around her on the pillow, Anne felt rested and more
like herself than she had for days. If only that
persistent, nagging pain would go away. She had just
jotted a few of her musings for the day and closed
her Journal when she heard Ben's footsteps down the
hall . . .

She quickly put her Journal aside and
straightened the covers.

He poked his head around the corner of the
bedroom doorway. "Good morning . . . uh, good
afternoon, Doctor Anne . . . are you ready for a tasty
repast?"

How young and boyish he looks, she thought,
but responded, "I'm famished, Ben. And I'm very,
very ready for your tasty repast."

How wan and weary she looks, he thought, but
said, "There's plenty for two, so I'll join you."

Their conversation was light and chatty.
Seemingly carefree. And *surface*, Ben thought. We
must talk. Soon. Today?

Chapter Thirteen

He looks so happy, Anne thought. Do I dare tell him about the biopsy today? But, if not today, when?

CHAPTER FOURTEEN

"Thank you for seeing me," Jack was saying.
They were seated in Dr. Diaz' mahogany-paneled
office. "North of the border cancer is mostly viewed as
the kiss of death, which, statistically it all too often
is. But down here . . ." he held his arms open wide
in a gesture of frustrated amazement. "And, well, I
just don't get it. Down here, it's different . . . I've got
to know why."

Diaz smiled warmly. "Things *are* different
down here. For one thing, our patients are living
longer. They often come in here on stretchers, unable
to walk, sometimes even unable to talk or care for
themselves . . ."

"And they walk out of here, Doctor? Is that
it?" Jack finished the sentence. "Is *that* the
difference?"

"Of course, it's not as simple as that. But,
speaking in a purely practical manner, that's right.
We don't save them all. Some are just too far gone.
They've been mutilated and scarred by what I call
primitive medicine . . ."

Jack winced. "You mean traditional, orthodox
medicine?"

"Yes. By the burning, cutting and poisoning
they've undergone."

"Surely, Dr. Diaz, you're not lumping all of
that, as you say, 'burning, cutting and poisoning' as
destructive?"

"Of course not. Some of the radiation and chemotherapy may be necessary. And surgery, especially surgery . . ."

"Please explain what you mean."

"I mean that some of the modalities you named *might* be useful, mostly as a purely emergency measure, so to speak, to buy the patient time. Time that will enable his or her own body to initiate the proper metabolic procedures that can halt the cancerous invasion and save his life . . .

"Sometimes . . ." Diaz continued, then paused, "sometimes, in fact, *often*, patients come to us as a last resort. I use the words last resort advisedly. But they have undergone surgery and radiation *and* chemotherapy to a point beyond which the body is able to rally its healing forces . . ."

He paused as though struggling for a descriptive term. "Yes, to a shameful degree. Perhaps *brutalized* would be a more accurate term. By the time they arrive at our doors, their bodies are debilitated and dehydrated, mere skin and bones, hardly able to function as human beings . . ."

"And at that point," Jack broke in cynically, "you perform your magic with laetrile." Leaning back in his chair, head cocked at an angle, with his arms crossed tightly against his chest, he could hardly have adopted a more defensive pose. Diaz was fully aware of Jack's negative body language, but chose to ignore the obvious challenge.

He smiled disarmingly and spoke softly. "Correction, Dr. Drury. We do not practice magic in our clinic. And laetrile is only part of our armamentarium . . ."

Jack smiled wryly. "Touche, Doctor. I am sorry. Please forgive me for the thrust."

Diaz nodded pleasantly. "Of course."

"But," Jack pressed, "what about tumors. Do you just ignore them and hope they'll go away? Do you cut them out? Do you treat them specifically in *any* way?"

"Good question, Doctor. For nearly thirty years our clinic has been treating cancers of all kind metabolically. We believe that all cancer is caused by a metabolic imbalance of some kind, so we . . ."

"Even tumors?" Jack interrupted.

"Especially tumors," Diaz went on smoothly, "While orthodox or traditional medicine continues to think of cancer as a *tumor*, and usually harmful, we recognize it as a *systemic condition*. We work on the thesis that lumps or bumps are merely *symptoms*, not the disease itself . . ."[13]

He paused for Jack's nod of understanding, then went on. "It's no wonder we doctors have failed to control cancer all these years. We, that is, generically, the profession as a whole, have been attacking the symptoms and ignoring the disease . . ."

Diaz' phone buzzed. He picked it up. "Rosalie, unless it's urgent, please hold my calls for another hour or so."

He turned back to Jack.

"We have learned that most tumors are a mixture of cancer cells and non-cancer cells. And, believe me, Doctor, it came as a shock when I learned that the greater portion of the average tumor is non-cancerous . . ."

"Yes," Jack said, "I realize that many researchers are beginning to say that."

Diaz smiled easily and went on. "Agreed. And though no one fully understands the mechanisms involved, apparently *the tumor actually is part of the body's defenses against cancer*."[14] He paused for emphasis, then continued.

"You see, when cancer begins to form, if the vitamin and pancreatic factors are insufficient to check it, the body, in its infinite wisdom, instigates an intelligent effort to save the life of the organism . . ."

"What are you saying, Doctor? That . . .?'"

"Exactly," Diaz said, speaking to the unspoken question, "in an heroic effort to seal off and isolate the cancer, the body surrounds it with millions of non-cancerous cells . . ."

"Wait a minute, Doctor! Hold it right there." Jack had raised both hands in a protective mode. "Let me get this clear. Are you saying that the body's healing mechanisms themselves actually *create* the tumor?"

"That's exactly what I'm saying. In a sense the tumor really is our 'friend' because it is attempting to save our life . . ."

"By preventing its cancerous contents from spreading to and through other parts of the body!" Jack broke in, comprehension beginning to dawn.

"Precisely, Doctor," Diaz said. "Precisely. Now, you've got the picture."

Jack slumped in his chair and slowly released the air from his lungs. His head was reeling. He had the odd sensation of having been levitated into another dimension, one in which he had no part, in which he did not belong. What he had just heard from Diaz undercut much of what he had been taught about cancer in med school . .

For the past six months, since first having made contact with the Mexican cancer clinics, Jack had been straining desperately to understand, to keep up with, and to integrate into his practice what he was trying to learn. Repeatedly he asked himself if the American medical profession could be wrong about alternative cancer research and treatment. And if it was wrong about that, what else?

His position, he thought, was comparable to attempting a tight wire balancing act. Behind him was the comfortable safety of orthodoxy. Before him the attractive uncertainties of alternative medicine. In the chasm beneath the sagging wire, clamoring for his attention, were the piteous faces and cries of thousands of nameless patients.

"What shall I do?" he asked Carolyn. "I'm no longer either a sheep or a goat. Neither a fish nor a fowl. I'm not a total allopathic physician . . . nor am I fully convinced of the efficacy of the alternative . . ."

She shook her head slowly. "Jack, I can't help you make up your mind. Nor should I. Literally, you're the doctor."

"But what would you do in my position?"

"I think I would carefully weigh the evidence. Then decide."

He groaned in frustration. "That's what I've been doing. For months . . . and I'm no closer to a decision than before."

They were driving back from Las Vegas in Jack's car where they had attended the Tri-State Holistic Convention. The night was sharp and clear with multitudes of stars sprinkled liberally across the heavens. Paradoxical with his emotional struggle, Jack was comfortably aware of Carolyn's female closeness and struggled to keep his mind upon his dilemma.

Carolyn had removed her shoes and curled her legs beneath her. She stretched sinuously, like a kitten, and in the dim reflection of the dash light he was aware of her sweater stretched tightly across her breasts.

She covered her mouth and yawned. "Why don't you visit Dr. Diaz . . . and talk to him?" she suggested, referring to the convention's keynote speaker, the head of a large cancer clinic in Tijuana. "You and he seemed to hit if off quite well."

"That's it!" Jack banged the wheel with his hand. "I should have thought of that. I'll do it. I've got his business card in my pocket. I'll telephone him tomorrow."

Now, two weeks later, seated in Diaz' office, the picture was beginning to clear itself.

"But I don't get it, Doctor . . ." Jack paused in confusion. "If all of this . . ." he waved his arms indicating the clinic, the concept itself, "if all of this that I see, all that you're telling me is true . . ."

Diaz nodded. "It's true."

"But, then, why . . .?"

"Why?" Diaz wrinkled his brows. "Why? Why what?"

"Why don't we practice this kind of medicine in the States? Why do we have to send patients to Mexico. Or to the Philippines? Or Germany? Or Greece? Or the Caribbean? Or, wherever? Why can't we do in the States what you're doing here?"

"Why?" Diaz' amazement at the question showed on his face.

"Yeah, Doctor. Why?" The harsh tone in his voice was a challenge.

"You ask why? As if you didn't already know the answer."

"I *don't* know the answer. I may suspect it. But . . ."

"Doctor, *could* you practice this kind of medicine in the United States? Or don't you choose to do so?"

"What are you talking about, Doctor?" Despite himself, an edge of anger crept into Jack's voice. "I *want* to practice this kind of medicine . . ."

Diaz smiled coldly. "Maybe you do, Doctor. Along with a few of your colleagues. But your government isn't with you in that regard. Neither are the medical and pharmaceutical monopolies.

"My question to you — and to them — is this: If what they have is so good, then why are they afraid to allow patients the freedom of choice? Because, if the therapies they are attempting to destroy aren't any good, they'll simply die of their own accord. That's just basic economics . . ."

He paused for effect. "But not even your father
. . . wants to practice this kind of medicine?"

"What do you mean?"

"Doctor, you know what I mean. Your father
kicked you out of his own clinic because you began to
stray from the fold . . ."

Amazement slid across Jack's face. "You know
about that?"

"Everybody in Los Angeles does. And in the
whole State of California." Diaz smiled sardonically.
"Your father's not exactly unknown. Nor are his
connections with the drug cartel . . ."

Jack winced. Drug cartel? His father? What
was Diaz talking about? These questions buzzed
around and around in his skull like a bee in a bottle,
but he said nothing. He was beginning to feel like a
culture on a microscope slide.

"Anyway," Diaz went on, "that's beside the
point . . ."

"Exactly what is the point?" Jack demanded.
Diaz' remarks were coming too close to home and
they rankled.

"The point is this: The United States refuses to
allow its citizens the freedom of medical choice their
own Constitution provides them . . ."

"Choice of *medical* freedom? What do you
mean?"

Diaz laughed harshly. "Have you read The Bill
of Rights to your Constitution lately?"

Jack squirmed uncomfortably. "No . . . no, I
guess not."

"Let me refresh your memory by quoting part
of it for you. 'No State shall make or enforce any law
which shall abridge the privileges or immunities of
citizens of the United States; nor shall any State
deprive any person of life, liberty, or property without
due process of law . . .'"[15]

When Diaz finished, Jack said, with some
embarrassment, "I guess I'd forgotten that . . ."

Diaz acknowledged Jack's admission with a nod. "During the same period of time," he went on, "Dr. Benjamin Rush, one of the signers of your Declaration of Independence — a medical doctor, by the way — made a very strong point.

"Dr. Rush told the leadership of your fledgling country, that the Constitution of the new Republic should make special provisions for *medical* freedom as well as religious freedom. He fervently believed that the art of healing should not be restricted to one class of men and denied to others. Such laws, he claimed, would be un-American and despotic."

When he finished speaking, Diaz clasped his hands together behind his head and leaned back in his leather chair. For a moment both men were lost in their thoughts.

"You shame me with my own ignorance . . ."

"Your country's Constitution guarantees you all sorts of freedoms, yet withholds many of them," Diaz stated flatly. "While Mexico guarantees those freedoms . . . and supports them. That's why I practice medicine down here."

"But, why shouldn't you practice medicine down here? You're a Mexican citizen . . ."

Diaz' voice sounded like ground glass. "That's true, I *am* a Mexican citizen . . . proud to be one. And I don't consider that to be a put down . . ."

"I didn't mean it that way . . ."

"Maybe. Maybe not. It's true, though, I was born in Mexico. I was educated in Mexico. I am a Mexican. But I am an excellent clinician."

Jack felt the blood rising in his face. "I didn't mean to imply . . ."

"You're an American, Doctor," Diaz went on evenly. "With your built-in gringo prejudice toward Mexicans. Everyone knows that's standard equipment."

He rose from behind his desk and stood in front of Jack. Though he was in total control of his emotions, it was apparent that he was angry.

Instinctively Jack backed away.

Diaz continued, his expression distinctly cool, his words clipped. "I told you I was educated in Mexico. That's true, but only partially true. I did all of my undergraduate work in Mexico. But, I earned my medical degree from the University of California in Los Angeles."

"So did my father," Jack responded quickly.

"I know," Diaz said. "I graduated the same year as your father — in the same class that he did . . ."

"I didn't realize . . ." Jack began.

Diaz went on, ignoring Jack's admission. "A fact I'm very much aware of." He went on silkily, tantalizingly, "Another fact: We sat in some of the same lecture halls together . . ."

"You did?"

"Yes, Doctor, we did. But he never knew I existed. Few Americans did. Why? Because I was a foreigner, a Mexican."

Jack's face burned. "I'm sorry," he said lamely.

Diaz shrugged and turned on his heel and strode back to his chair behind his desk. Neither man spoke for a few moments.

"Look, Doctor," Diaz began, his voice now mellow, elbows upon his desk, "I've got all the credentials I need to practice medicine in the United States, or anywhere else in the world that I want to practice."

He indicated the wall behind him which was liberally covered with a panoply of degrees, diplomas, awards and commendations. And photographs. One of Diaz smilingly accepting a rolled scroll, two others, apparently receiving awards of some kind, from former American presidents. Yet other photographs depicting awards being heaped upon a capped and

157

gowned Diaz from dignitaries in obvious educational settings.

Despite himself, Jack was impressed and said so.

Diaz nodded acceptance. "Doctor, I practice medicine in Mexico for two reasons. We've already discussed the first one."

He paused. Jack accepted the cue. "And the other one?"

"Because my modis operandi displeased the cartel . . ."

"The cartel?"

"Yes. The medical/pharmaceutical cartel. They made it plain to me that my presence would be more tolerable elsewhere. Pronto! The sooner the better." He grinned coldly. "So I left. Pronto!"

Jack Drury's mind was in a whirl. He had heard such stories before, of certain officials "requesting" that doctors either change their methods or change their locale. But this was the first time he'd come face to face with such a victim. Without a doubt Diaz was well educated. His diplomas attested to that. By his own admission he was a good clinician. Besides, the man's record spoke for itself. As did scores and hundreds of patients who attested to the man's skill.

Absentmindedly Jack watched the sun's rays slide across Diaz' face, giving it for a moment the appearance of stern, chiselled stone. He sighed.

"Dr. Diaz, I apologize . . ."

Diaz smiled expansively. "Why? Not necessary. My skin — as you Americanos say — is tough. My shoulders are broad . . ."

Jack shook his head. "I've been behaving like a typical ugly, arrogant American. And I'm sorry. I hope you will forgive me . . ." He arose.

Diaz rose also and moved quickly around the desk. "But, of course. Nothing to forgive. Misunderstanding." He shrugged.

Jack stuck out his hand. "You're kind and generous, Doctor. I have much to learn . . . from you. From others." He grimaced, "Whether Mexican or American."

Diaz chuckled. "We all have much to learn . . . I will be glad to share with you. Anything we are doing here. *Everything* we are doing here. It's all available to you. To the public. To the world . . ."

Jack gripped Diaz' hand. "And, Doctor, as I've learned, the price is right. *Very* right."

"Thank you, amigo."

"May I come back?"

"Of course. Any time. You are always welcome . . ."

Sunday afternoon was merging with evening as Drury, along with many thousands of other Americanos lined up to recross the border into California. In the exhaust-filled atmosphere, as Jack laboriously jockeyed his car toward the Customs booth, he had a great deal to mull over in his mind.

Uppermost was the persistent question, *Why do so few Americans fail to avail themselves of this lifesaving expertise?*

Comfortably ensconced in the deck chairs of their hilltop retreat, where they had just watched the sun reluctantly dip below the ocean rim, leaving behind it a glorious sunset, Ben Rush was asking his wife the same question.

CHAPTER FIFTEEN

"It has never become easy for me to tell a patient, or a patient's spouse what I'm going to tell you," Dr. Cranston was saying. He was sitting on the corner of the huge desk that dwarfed his tiny office.

Seated, with both his feet planted firmly on the floor, Ben gripped his knees with his hands to keep them from shaking. He swallowed, but didn't answer.

Cranston spoke softly, almost gently. "Dr. Rush, your wife, is a valued colleague and an excellent clinician . . . but she is also a very sick woman . . ."

Nothing in Ben's previous experience prepared him for the horror of the next few months. Two weeks after Dr. Cranston took Anne's biopsy, his office had telephoned. Anne wasn't home at the time, so Ben took the call.

"Hello. Ben Rush . . ."

The nurse identified herself, then proceeded to inform Ben that "Dr. Cranston has made arrangements for Dr. Rush's surgery tomorrow morning. He has secured her hospital room. And in order to adequately prep her for surgery, your wife should arrive at the hospital some time this evening and be . . ."

"Wait a minute!" Ben almost shouted in the telephone. "What do you mean, 'Dr. Rush's surgery?'

There must be some mistake. What surgery are you talking about?"

The startled nurse responded that she was only relaying Dr. Cranston's instructions. His hands and voice trembling, Ben said, "We've made no arrangements for surgery. We haven't even heard the results of the biopsy . . ."

There was a long silence at the other end of the line.

"Hello," Ben insisted. "Talk to me. Tell me what's going on. I want to know what's happening."

"I can only repeat what I have already told you . . ." the nurse began, "which is that Dr. Cranston . . ."

"Hold it right there," Ben commanded. "I know you're not at fault. But Dr. Rush is my wife. What's happening here concerns me as well as her. May I please speak with Dr. Cranston . . ."

Obviously shaken by this turn of events, the nurse indicated that the doctor was with a patient at the moment, but that she would have him call Mr. Rush back. Ben thanked her and hung up. A deep mantle of apprehensive gloom descended across his shoulders and he felt weighted down with despair.

He paced the floor of his office like a caged lion. Twice he reached for the telephone to call Anne, but changed his mind. No, he could not call her at the clinic. Suddenly he became aware of a truth so obvious that he wondered he hadn't seen it before. *Anne knew how ill she was. She knew!*

And she was trying to spare him by hiding it from him.

"Oh, God . . . oh, God . . ." He dropped to his knees beside his chair and pressed his forehead against the cool leather seat.

The telephone's shrilling started him. He climbed to his feet and caught it on the first ring. "Yes. Ben Rush."

"Please hold for Dr. Cranston . . ." The line became silent.

Ben clutched the phone till his fingers ached.

In a moment he heard, "Mr. Rush, this is Dr. Cranston. Are there any questions I can answer for you?"

"Yes, Doctor. Your nurse spoke of my wife's surgery . . ." With an effort he kept his voice under control. "I didn't know what she was talking about. Surgery? What for?"

Cooly distant and professional, Cranston said, "Mr. Rush, as I am assuming you know, we did a biopsy on you wife. That is, we took a piece of tissue . . ."

"Dr. Cranston, I *know* what a biopsy is. What I *don't* know is the results, the report of that biopsy. Nor do I know anything of the surgery that you apparently have scheduled for my wife. The surgery that we — at least I — know nothing about!"

After a brief hesitation, Cranston indicated that his office had mailed the report to the Rush's home address nearly a week ago by Certified mail. "The receipt came back this morning, Mr. Rush. So I naturally assumed that you knew . . ."

It came to him now, Anne's strangely restless behavior the past few days. Her sleepless nights. Dark circles under her eyes in the mornings. The haunted look upon her face. How she had started to speak to him a few times, but then had stopped in mid-sentence. Yes, Anne knew. But had been reluctant to tell him.

"Oh, my God, Doctor. I guess . . . I mean, I don't know quite what to say . . ."

The doctor's voice was instantly warm with understanding. "Mr. Rush, something of this nature is difficult to share with one you love . . ."

Apprehension gripped him again. "Dr. Cranston, what do you mean by 'something of this nature'? Tell me. Please."

He heard the doctor draw a deep breath and let it out. "I think you should come to my office so we can talk."

"When?"

"How about right now. How long will it take you to get to my office? Twenty minutes or so?"

"Yes, Doctor. I can leave right this minute . . ."

Now, seated in Cranston's cramped office, he was hearing the words of doom that he now realized Anne already knew. "In addition to the biopsy, Mr. Rush, we also did a computerized axial tomography, a CAT scan, on your wife . . ."

He paused and Ben shrugged.

"The scan indicated a number of enlarged abdominal lymph nodes . . . attached to the aorta. They were quite large — up to 2.2 centimeters in diameter . . ."

He paused again and checked Anne's chart.

Ben forced himself to ask, "Exactly what does that mean?"

Cranston removed his glasses and slid them into the pocket of his white coat. "Both the enlarged nodes and the spleen were consistent with a diagnosis of lymphoma."

He stopped talking and waited for Ben's response.

"Lymphoma. That's cancer . . . of the lymph glands?"

"To put it simply, yes."

"Which means the . . . lymphoma . . . the cancer . . . has already spread . . . throughout the body . . .?"

Cranston nodded. "Yes, metastasized is the medical term." He rose and moved to the window and leaned against the ledge facing Ben. "However, Ben . . . it *may not* be too late . . . at least to buy some time . . . with surgery and chemotherapy."

Ben shuddered. "Surgery *and* chemotherapy? That's horrible!"

"Yes, I know . . ." Cranston whispered. "How well I know."

Ben gripped his knees till they screamed in concert with his agonized spirit. "Doctor, isn't there . . ." he croaked, "isn't there . . . *any* recourse?"

Cranston didn't speak. He slowly shook his head.

That day had initiated Ben's chamber of horrors. The rest had been a jumble of nightmares. How he negotiated his way home through the congested traffic without an accident was a mystery Ben didn't consider till later. But when he arrived at their condo in Santa Monica, he realized he had absolutely no memory of the drive from Cranston's office.

Anne's car was in her stall.

He stumbled upstairs and entered.

Anne, looking like a pale ghost, met him and wordlessly fell into his arms. The look on his face told her everything. Neither spoke. Finally, Ben led her to the living room and seated her in front of the fireplace. He had laid the fire earlier. Now he touched a match and welcomed the warm glow . . .

Impulsively he fell to his knees beside his wife and dropped his head in her lap. Suddenly the dam broke, and the pent up fears of the past weeks and months forced themselves from his system . . .

Anne had done her bitter weeping during the nights as he had slept. Now she lovingly caressed her husband's head and hair as the warm, gentle tears trickled down her cheeks.

They spoke little. There was no need.

Later, as Anne moved about packing her small case for the hospital, Ben sat still, his eyes feasting upon her every move. As though this domestic scene might never be reenacted.

Dr. Anne's Journal

Immensely satisfied with himself, Roger Keller accepted the champagne from the 747 First Class cabin attendant. The bubbly liquid served only to enhance his euphoria. He twirled the slender-stemmed glass in his pudgy fingers. "I have done it," he chortled to himself. "I have achieved the impossible!"

"A little more, Mr. Keller?" the smiling hostess offered.

He waved her away with a predatory gleam. "Later, perhaps?"

Though in her early thirties, the young woman was an airline veteran. She flashed him a bright-toothed smile and coquettishly parried his thrust. "Perhaps?"

His Don Juan advances properly acknowledged, Keller wriggled his bulky derriere more deeply into the luxurious lounge chair, propped up his bootie-clad feet, and slid the thin folder from his crocodile-skin attache case.

Already enormously wealthy and powerful, this latest product would jet-propel Bullion, Inc., International, into a position eons beyond its closest competitors, and guarantee a place of eminence in the pharmaceutical world that could never be surpassed. And for him — Roger Keller, BII's CEO and chairman of the Board of Directors — a place in the sun that could never be eclipsed.

It was a deeply satisfied man who opened the thin folder to the first page . . .

As with every pharmaceutical company, progress is cyclical, and not every year, hardly any given decade, resulted in the development of a new product or products that would keep them in the forefront of the industry, hence the public eye.

And — consequently — that would reap for the company the high profits they believed they deserved.

At any one time BII employed over 200 research chemists and other researchers, and though involved in a variety of different projects, the focus for all was the same: Discover new, lucrative products, and/or perfect and/or modify existing products so as to dynamically increase the company's income.

All too often the profit motive superseded the eleemosynary goal projected by the company image.

With few exceptions, each of those 200 plus researchers hoped to be the one who would hit upon that magical formula or compound that would blast them out of the mediocrity of their existence into the limelight of praise and monetary reward.

Judine Kelso was one of those exceptions.

Though young for her notable list of accomplishments, Judine had a vested goal of her own. Or, rather, a dual goal: one, to justify her uncle's faith in her. And, two, to forever wipe out and destroy the power of pain upon cancer victims.

As a young teenager, Judine had been forced to sit idly by and watch her widowed mother succumb to the ravages of cancer. At the last the woman's pain had been so intense that not even the heaviest allowable drugs could dull her agony. Judine's emotional pain teetered on the edge, and when her mother finally breathed her last, Judine's resolve snapped and she went berserk.

Before the girl could be subdued and straight jacketed by four male orderlies, Judine had made a. shambles of her mother's hospital room. With nowhere to go and no place to turn, it was her mother's brother who took the girl under his wing. He raised her in his own home and educated her at his own expense.

Dr. Anne's Journal

Judine never forgot. She plowed through her undergraduate, master's and doctoral programs till she earned the Ph.D. degree in Oncological Chemistry, magna cum laude. She applied to Bullion for a position as a research assistant and was hired immediately.

The man who placed Judine on BII's payroll was her uncle, Roger Keller. Intuitively he believed she could be the key to his own ultimate future. Five years later, he had put Judine under his own wing. Since that time, she had reported to him only.

Most oncological research scientists are quite naturally bent upon seeking a cure for cancer, the most dreaded of all diseases, one responsible for the deaths of one-half million Americans annually. Not Judine. Though she kept her innermost feelings on the subject to herself, she did not believe that a cure for cancer existed.

She sought only a means of ameliorating the unbearable agonies experienced by many terminal patients. If, however, in the process, as BII and Roger Keller hoped, she were to perfect a cure for cancer, that would be a bonus. But Judine herself was not seeking it.

One month ago Judine completed her 10th year at BII, the last five under Keller's tutelage. With Keller's full knowledge and authority, Judine had focused the majority of those five years on a project of her own design and choice, known only to herself and to him. Her lab notes and records referred to the project by the unimaginative title: 8590-983. That name was only for the books..

Between Roger Keller and herself, the product was referred to as Oncoplex.

Judine knew that chemotherapy regimens were usually composed of several drugs, referred to by an acronym arranged from the names of those drugs. CHOP was one of the more commonly used chemotherapy regimens, which was composed of cyclophosphamide, hydroxydaunomycin, Oncovin and prednisone. Such compounds, Judine knew, were harsh, caustic, and generally at least as detrimental to the health of the patients as they were to the cancer cells they were intended to eliminate.

What Judine had been attempting was to perfect a formula that would combine all the best attributes of several such drugs and utilize it on patients as a single drug. Such a drug, she believed, would avoid the harsher aspects of chemotherapy while still providing the expected benefits.

However, as so often happens in research, the project took on a life of its own. Intrigued, Judine decided to follow this new bent, at least for a while. But to her amazement, she arrived at a totally unexpected and different destination than the one she anticipated. Instead of isolating a drug compound that would *kill*, or at least cripple the cancer cells, thus giving the body the strength to fight, she had stumbled upon a drug that would *prevent* cancer cells from finding refuge in the body.

She conducted her experiments on mice. Time and again she repeated her series, checked her protocol and figures, only to arrive at the same conclusions. She longed to share her discovery with other scientists, but dared not. Oncoplex's potential value was of such magnitude that an information leak could sabotage the entire project.

Though Judine was by now a somewhat seasoned scientist, she found herself becoming more excited than she had ever been. If she was correct in her protocols and conclusions — and she saw no possible flaw in her computations — she knew that Oncoplex would have breathtaking implications for the entire drug world.

Judine allowed herself an extra month during which to check and recheck every step, every experiment, each bit of data. The results were decisive. Precise. Unchallengeable. But with a new, bonus benefit she had not anticipated, almost more important than the one she had first discovered.

Today was the day, Judine decided, to reveal to Roger Keller the fullness of her discovery. With trembling fingers she dialed his private number.

"Yes," he answered, knowing it must be she.

Despite her effort to remain cool, her words rushed out in a breathless tumble. "I've got to talk to you . . ."

By now he knew her too well to deny her an audience. Knowing that she was single minded and almost totally unfrivolous, he did not hesitate. "When?"

"Now. Some time today." The excitement in her voice was evident.

"Where?"

"In my lab?"

He checked his appointments. "I can be there in an hour."

Forty-five minutes later he rapped at her door. She knew he was too busy a man to waste time. She got right to the point. "I believe you understand the trophoblast theory?"

He nodded impatiently. "Of course. Otherwise known as the Unitarian Trophoblast Thesis?"

"Yes."

She opened her book. "Look at this . . ."

He read rapidly, skimming her notes with comprehension. As he read, Judine watched him, noted the pulse quicken in his neck, the increased respiration, the bead of perspiration form on his forehead. Five minutes later he looked up, attempting to disguise his evident excitement.

He asked a simple question. "Are you certain?"

"Yes. There's no doubt about it."

"Judine, are you telling me that Oncoplex *prevents* cancer cells from finding a refuge, a home, in the body?"

"That's correct. But that's not all . . ."

He held up his hand. "Are you further telling me that this drug you've been working on, Oncoplex, is also a contraceptive?"

She nodded. "Yes."

He frowned. "Judine, think carefully. I want to be certain I'm hearing what I think I'm hearing. Are you telling me that Oncoplex not only prevents cancer cells from finding and retaining a foothold in the body, but that it also prevents the fertilization of the ovum?"

"You've got it partially right. Oncoplex does prevent cancer cells from fastening themselves to a fixed location. But it does not prevent the sperm from fertilizing the ovum. However, it does something that is every bit as important: It prevents the fertilized ovum from attaching itself to the wall of the uterus. And by so doing, the fertilized, but unattached ovum, remains unattached, and is thus flushed out of the woman's system."

"For all intents and purposes, then, a contraceptive?"

Judine nodded. "That's correct. You've got the picture."

Roger sat down weakly. "Fantastic. Fantastic!"

"There's more. Oncoplex is better than the Pill. It doesn't poison the body. It does not kill cells, cancer or otherwise. All it does is prevent the cancer cells from setting up shop, so to speak, in one location, and proliferating. That's all."

He whistled.

"Run that by me again."

"Okay. A fertilized egg is a trophoblast cell, sometimes referred to as a totipotent stem cell. It attaches itself to the wall of the uterus and begins growing at an incredible rate, doubling in size every few minutes until it finally becomes a fetus . . ."

"Okay. Okay, Judine, I've got that. Go on."

"Okay, according to the Trophoblast Theory, the Unitarian Theory, a cancer cell and a fertilized ovum are identical in makeup. And the cancer cell, precisely like the fertilized ovum, also grows and multiplies at an incredible rate . . ."

"You are telling me that for all practical purposes, the fertilized ovum and the cancer cell are alike?"

Judine nodded.

"Therefore, if Oncoplex prevents cancer cells from attaching themselves someplace, as it does the fertilized ovum, the body will reject and eliminate them. Is that it?"

"You've got it. That's it."

"And you've tested it . . . thoroughly?"

"Thoroughly. Here are all of my records. They're impeccable."

A crafty look crept into Roger's eyes. "Does anyone else know of your research?"

"Nobody. Nobody has the slightest idea what I've been doing."

He indicated her notebooks. "These are the only copies?"

"That's right. There are no others."

He spoke with growing excitement. "Where do you keep them?"

"Locked up in my safe. Only you and I have the combination."

That was only yesterday. Now, high over the Atlantic, Roger feasted upon Judine's summaries. Information, he knew, that if it was accurate, would shake the entire world. And if Bullion, or he, Roger Keller, were able to harness this information, it would enable the owner quite literally, to control the world.

Keller closed his eyes and visualized the almost total raw power such a product could command. Suddenly his eyes snapped open wide. There was only one thing that could possibly hinder the success of Oncoplex: the lobbying efforts of the so-called freedom of medical choice movement through men like Dr. Sidney Wolfe[16]; Maureen Salaman, Clinton and Bonnie Miller[17]; and others[18] such as Ralph Nader . . .

And muckrakers like Mike Culbert in that infernal *Choice* Magazine[19]. If they were all to unite and push for more extensive testing of Oncolplex, it could delay the introduction of the product. And the cost would soar to prohibitive figures.

Something had to be done about them. All of them!

He quickly flipped his seat upright, unbuckled himself and located a radiotelephone. Slipping in his credit card, he dialed a secret number. Five thousand miles away, Bertram Collins excused himself from a client and picked up the line reserved exclusively for Keller. "Yes?" he said.

Without preamble, Keller spoke softly, "I've got what I need. It's time to move. Put the plan into action . . ."

Collins listened intently to Keller's instructions, taking no notes. When Keller finished, Collins nodded. "Right," he said. "Consider it done . . ."

Before returning to his client, he buzzed his secretary. "Get hold of Drury . . . and my daughter. I want to talk to each of them. Separately. Interrupt me as soon as you get either one of them on the line . . ."

CHAPTER SIXTEEN

Allen Drury sat slumped at his desk, trembling violently. The silent telephone stared mockingly at him. Bertram Collins had reached him on the freeway via cellular on his way to his office. Typical of the man, he'd had begun speaking without introduction, "Call me back in twenty minutes . . ."

At his office, minutes before eight, Drury dialed Collins' unlisted number.

Again, without preamble, "Have you gotten to Jack yet?"

Allen felt sweat begin sliding down his back. "I've tried."

"Not good enough, Al. Trying won't get you anything. Get to him. Now. Today."

"Okay, Bert. But, what's the rush?"

"Things are coming down, Al. The pressure's on. We've got to prevent any health professionals — the ones people will believe, you know, the ones with solid medical backgrounds — we've got to keep them from giving any credence to what the alternative boys are saying. Understand?"

Allen sighed. "Okay, Bert . . ."

"What about Anne?" Collins demanded.

"Anne? She's in the hospital. Surgery. Cancer surgery. Now. This morning."

At that precise moment, walking stocking-footed down the hallway, with her driving shoes in her hand, Carolyn was about to pass Drury's office door. The mention of Anne's name caught her attention and she stopped to listen. Who was Drury talking to?

Carolyn's heart pounded. Anne? Hospital? Surgery? Why hadn't she said something? No wonder she had been so jumpy and distracted yesterday . . .

For the briefest moment Collins paused. When he spoke again Drury didn't notice the slightest tremor of feeling or emotion.

"Oh . . . she was telling me she had cancer of some kind. Right now that's beside the point. The point is this: Keep Jack away from her!"

"What do you mean, keep Jack away from Anne? That doesn't make sense. They scarcely know each other."

"Keep it that way. Understand? I don't want Anne to get mixed up with any of that alternative quack medicine. Especially now . . ."

"Bert, Anne's your daughter. She needs all the help she can get. And alternative medicine isn't going to harm her . . ."

"Just the same, keep her out of it. Out of the way. Got it? I don't want her to have anything to do with them."

"Yes, I understand." Drury pulled out a handkerchief and mopped his perspiring brow.

"There's a lot coming down. And you can help keep your name clean if you keep Jack out of this. Because, if those alternative boys get in the way, they'll be getting hurt . . .

"Okay, Bert . . . okay. I'll hold up my end here."

With a start, Carolyn realized that Drury had been talking to Anne's father, the San Francisco attorney. But why didn't he want her involved with alternative medicine? If she had lymphoma, that might be the best thing for her . . .

By now Carolyn knew she'd heard too much. Tiptoeing back to the entrance, she slipped on her shoes and walked normally along the hallway. When she passed Drury's doorway she realized that her subterfuge was unnecessary. Drury was slumped at his desk, staring dumbly at the telephone in his hand . . .

Carolyn hurried to her desk and set her things down. Keeping an eye on Drury's office door, she dialed Anne's number. It rang until the electronic answering device came on. She replaced the instrument and hurriedly dialed another familiar number.

Jack's pleasant voice answered with a cheerful, "Good morning!"

Cupping her hand over the mouthpiece she spoke softly. "Jack, we've got to talk. Very important. No . . . not now. No, I can't tell you what it's about. Lunch? Fine . . . see you then."

CHAPTER SEVENTEEN

A huge fire roared in the fireplace of the Malibu cabin. Ben poured himself a glass of apple juice and set it on the hearth. He seated himself comfortably in his chair, and adjusted his lapboard, painfully aware of the vacant chair opposite him. All day long he'd been puttering around the cabin, as though to avoid this moment.

Finally, with all other preparations in order, he picked up the battered, leather-bound volume and opened it to Anne's final entry . . .

> *May 15, 4:30 a.m. — To you, Ben, my dear, darling husband. You must know by now how very much I love you . . .*
>
> *Please don't grieve for me. I will never leave you. My spirit will be with you always. A favor I ask: Please complete the work that I have begun. You will find every detail faithfully recorded. But, Ben, do more than I did. Search out the whole truth and expose it. I now believe that I did not have to die of cancer. But, I did not know it soon enough. Nor was I strong enough to resist the forces that forged the chains of fear upon me. I will be with you always . . . forever . . .*

Dr. Anne's Journal

The last entry was not signed . . .

The St. John's Hospital waiting room was crowded, the air heavy with the sour, stale odor of controlled panic. Ben had brought a manuscript to edit, but spent most of his time pacing the marble corridors and checking the tortoise-slow movement of the dragging minutes . . . and hours.

Eschewing conversation, he avoided all those who endeavored to waylay him and distract him from his tortured vigil.

Anne had been scheduled for surgery at six. Ben was in her room by five as the nurses began prepping her for surgery. How tiny, how fragile she looked. When the orderlies came with the gurney, she clung to him . . .

"Don't go away . . . please?"

He smiled tightly, hoping he didn't look as grim as he felt. "They couldn't drive me away, my dear, Doctor Anne. I will be *with you* through it all . . . and in your room when you return."

That had been three hours ago!

What could they be doing to her?

He ground his knuckles into his forehead to ease the throbbing that consumed his head . . .

"Ben . . . Ben . . ."

He looked up. It was Cranston, still in his green surgery gown, mask slipped down around his chin. He jumped up, spilling pages of his manuscript across the tile floor.

"Yes, Doctor. How . . . how did it go? How is she?"

Cranston was not smiling. He gripped Ben's elbow in his powerful hand. "Sit down, Ben . . ."

A white-hot knife sliced through Ben's heart.

"We did the best we could do . . . the very best . . ." He paused, his eyes sad.

"And . . .?" Ben rasped through his suddenly sandpapery throat. "How . . .?"

Cranston shook his head. "I don't know. I honestly don't know. We did the very best we could do . . ." The man's eyes bore mute tribute to his weariness. "It's out of my hands now . . ."

He closed his eyes. Ben sat very still. Curiously he noted his hands throbbing in resonance with his heart. He became acutely aware of the anesthetic odor of Dr. Cranston's clothing . . .

"It's times like these . . ." Cranston was musing, more to himself than to Ben, "when I am awed by the marvelous wonder of the human body . . . and the human spirit . . ."

He stretched out his hands and viewed them as though they belonged to another. "Yet, all the accumulated skill of a lifetime cannot perform miracles. Only God can do that . . ."

He sighed heavily.

Ben's insides turned to ice. "Then . . . she . . . I mean?" He couldn't finish the question.

Cranston struggled to his feet. He put his arms around Ben and held him tightly. "Go and be with Anne, my boy. She needs you. They'll be returning her to her room by now."

Leaving Ben's questions unanswered, Cranston turned and lumbered away, his head down.

Ben blindly gathered up his spilled manuscript and stuffed them into his attache case. As he headed for the elevator, he had the weird sense that he had been this way before . . .

Ben tossed another log on the fire and stirred the embers till the fire blazed. He pulled a blanket over his legs and continued to read . . .

Time and again an anguished groan forced itself from the depths of his burdened, lonely spirit. Anne . . . oh, Anne. Why didn't I know more? Why couldn't you have told me?

Twice he threw the blanket aside and strode out into the dark night. "Why . . . why did they do it to her? Why couldn't they have left her alone?" he screamed into the darkness. A coyote's eerie, high-pitched howl seemed to match his own frustration.

In agony of spirit Ben headed down the long driveway at a fast pace that soon became a trot. Before he reached the bottom of the hill he was jogging recklessly, till his heart threatened to beat its way out of his body and his breath came in long, rasping gasps.

He was still panting heavily when he again seated himself before the fire and took up the Journal . . .

The tip of the golden sun cleared the distant mountain as he turned to the last page and read again Anne's farewell. He laid the Journal on his lap and absentmindedly caressed its smooth patina. His mind whirled, clicked, whirled again. One by one the cogs began falling into place.

Reading Anne's Journal had its cathartic effect . . .

He felt cleansed . . .

Motivated . . .

And for the first time since she had gone, Ben knew exactly what he would do with the rest of his life . . .

CHAPTER EIGHTEEN

Sleep was a long time coming that night. The bed was empty. The cabin was pregnant with silence. He found himself listening for *her* noises: her humming or singing in the kitchen or shower. The clacking of her typewriter. Her voice on the telephone . . .

But now . . .

Had he allowed it, he could have visualized the future as bleak and empty. That was not his way. Nor Anne's. In her Journal she had plotted a course for him to follow.

Not an easy course. Nor straight. Rather a course fraught with convolutions, mazes and blind alleys. One-way streets and cul-de-sacs. Pitfalls, ambushes and booby traps.

Ben knew what he must do, but shrunk from it. By nature warm and gregarious, he generally found it easy and pleasurable to dialogue with people. Confrontations bothered him. But the road he must take, if he was to vindicate Anne's untimely demise, would include research, hard, grubby, time-consuming, tedious research . . .

Possibly even dangerous.

It would also include confrontations. Confrontations with individuals and entities, whose goals did not coincide with the best interests: the health and aspirations, indeed, even the *wellness* or happiness of fellow travellers.

Dr. Anne's Journal

The night before Ben had thoroughly read Anne's Journal. Today he *studied* it. He took copious notes. Listed names, addresses and telephone numbers. He noted dates and places of meetings. The agendas of such meetings, participants and their specific conversations.

More than once he resorted to Annes' medical library for definitions of terms and clarifications of concepts, marvelling as he did, at the breadth and understanding, the intelligent grasp of the subject matter recorded and discussed by Anne. He carefully recorded names of patients, the descriptions of their complaints or ailments, the diagnoses made, protocols utilized in treatment, and by whom. And each prognosis.

He often paused to stare — unseeingly — at the broad, unfettered sweeps of the Pacific . . . Time and again he raised his voice in anger: at individuals and the systems they represented. Then return his attention to the business at hand.

In the late afternoon, he unlocked Anne's Mercedes and slid into the driver's seat. He had gotten her this car when his first book had hit the *New York Times* best-seller list. Though it hadn't been driven for two years, it started immediately. He revved up the engine, checked all systems, then drove it to Point Dume.

There he stopped at the Last Resort Print Shop, the hardware store, Mayfair Market and the Post Office.

An hour later he was home again. Determined to complete the task he had begun, Ben worked steadily for several more hours. The sun had long since set before he was finished. He relaxed himself with a hot shower, then prepared and ate his simple evening meal.

He smiled at Anne's picture on the dresser. "Dear Doctor Anne . . . we got started on our project today . . ." In the dim light it seemed that she smiled in approval.

A plan in mind and a way to implement it determined, Ben slept deeply that night. Tomorrow morning he would make a visit to Cutting Edge and Ross Hannibal . . .

"I'll have one of your famous Idaho russet potatoes," Ben told the waiter, "the one that's baked in clay . . ."

"Anything else?"

"Just the salad bar. It looks especially good today."

Hannibal chuckled, "Sea Lion specials. Along with the excellent fish they serve here, their baked potatoes and salads are the best in the West." He spoke to the waiter. "Make mine the same . . ."

Though the hot, desert, Santa Ana winds were blowing, and the entire Los Angeles region was experiencing one of the hottest summers on record, Malibu Sea Lion was comfortably cool.

Hannibal suggested, "Agreeable that we visit the salad bar before we talk?"

"Okay by me . . ."

"Well, Ross, I am ready to start the project," Ben said when they were back at their seats.

"Good, I thought you might be," the editor said. He forked a juicy cherry tomato into his mouth, then reached into his attache case. ". . . so I took the liberty of bringing a contract . . ."

They discussed publishing policies while they ate. When the waiter cleared the table, Hannibal began, "I suppose you've got a plan of action?"

Ben fingered the unread contract. "Mind if I run this by my attorney?"

"I'd like you to. It's basically standard, though I beefed it up some . . . travel allowance. Secretarial. A few other items to make the job flow better. And faster."

"Thanks," Ben said and slipped the contract into his jacket pocket. "And to answer your question, yes, I do have a plan. At least a skeleton plan."

"Share it with me," Hannibal said, pulling out his ever present yellow lined pad.

"Although I was married to a doctor," Ben began, "I think it's obvious that I'm not a doctor, nor extremely knowledgeable in the medical field . . ."

Hannibal nodded.

"But I read a lot. And I live a fairly healthy lifestyle. So I'm not totally ignorant in the health field. But, Ross, after reading Anne's journal . . ." he patted his brief case.

". . . and I read every word of it yesterday. Some of it I read several times. But, after that, I not only believe that my wife died unnecessarily, but that a high percentage of the half million Americans who die of cancer each year die needlessly."

He paused and looked to Hannibal for affirmation. Hannibal merely nodded and said, "Go on . . ."

"Okay. Ross, I am convinced that . . ." he stopped in mid-sentence. "Do you know who the original Benjamin Rush was? The man I was named after?"

"Sure. *Dr*. Benjamin Rush — he was a medical doctor — and was the Physician General of the Middle Department of the Continental Army in 1777."[20]

Ben grinned in admiration. "Good. Very good! Anything else?"

"Yes. He was also one of the signers of the Declaration of Independence . . ."

"Right," Ben said, "and I'm proud to figure him somewhere in my family tree. Anyway, during those very troubled times, Dr. Rush strongly believed and preached that the Constitution of this Republic should make special provisions for *medical* freedom as well as religious freedom. To fail to do that, he said, would be un-American and despotic . . ."

Hannibal shook his head. "A strong statement."

"Exactly. And, Ross, I firmly believe that many of those people who die of cancer each year do so for one reason . . ."

"Which is?" Hannibal prompted.

"Because they don't have medical freedom of choice! The treatments, alternative treatments that *are available* — well-researched, well-documented modalities, modalities that can be had in the Philippines, in Greece, and other countries, one of them just across our southern border in Mexico — are simply not allowed here in the United States!"

Ben slammed his fist on the table. "And, Ross, that's not the kind of freedom that's guaranteed to us by Article Nine of the Bill of Rights. And it's a travesty. It's wrong. Wrong!"

Hannibal was solemnly shaking his head. He reached across the table and momentarily gripped Ben's two hands with his own. "Ben, you are right. The system is wrong. We both know that. But . . . now that you know it . . . what are *you* going to do about it?"

Overcome with emotion, Ben stared out across the sparkling Pacific . . . *pacific*, he thought. It means peaceful. But I feel anything but peaceful right now . . .

Finally he turned back to Hannibal, the fire of purpose burning in his eyes. "I'll tell you what I want to do . . . and I will, if Cutting Edge will back me . . . I want to inform the American public — and the entire world — that there are *many* options for dealing with cancer. Safe and tested ways that don't harm the body and destroy the immune system. And to communicate that information directly to the people, so they'll be able to avail themselves of those life-giving options."

He placed both hands flat upon the table. His intensely brown eyes bored into Hannibal's. "That's what I want to do, Ross . . . and, so help me, God, I believe I can do it."

Emotionally exhausted, Ben slumped back in his seat.

"Let me assure you of two things," Hannibal began, "no, three. First, I agree with you 100 percent. Second, I believe you can do the job you have outlined . . . and . . ." He paused and closed his lips.

"And the third one?" Ben asked.

"Speaking for Cutting Edge," Hannibal said softly, "they have given me the authority to tell you that *we will back you all the way*. Go to it. We're behind you!"

"Doctor's office," Carolyn said for what seemed the fiftieth time the past hour. "Dr. Drury? May I tell him who's calling?"

She gasped. "Mr. Rush . . . oh, my. Are you . . .?"

"Yes," Ben said softly, "I am Ben Rush, husband of the late Anne Rush . . ." He said it evenly, unsuccessfully repressing the emotion he felt.

Carolyn's words poured out. "Oh, Mr. Rush . . . I am so, so terribly sorry . . . I mean . . ."

"Thank you, Miss . . ."

"Kemp. Carolyn Kemp . . ."

"Anne, that is, Dr. Rush, thought of you as her friend. She spoke of you often."

With an effort Carolyn controlled herself. "Thank you. I, well, I really admired her. She was a wonderful doctor . . ."

"Thank you . . ."

Carolyn went on, "Well, uh, Mr. Rush, Dr. Drury is with a patient just now. Would you like him to return the call?"

"Not really," Ben said. "I really would like to set up an appointment. Not a medical appointment. I just want to talk with him . . ." Before Carolyn could respond, he added, "and with you. I'd like to talk with you, too. Not in the office . . ."

Carolyn caught her breath, but answered evenly, "I will tell Dr. Drury about your request, and he will be getting back to you. As for me — well, I'd be happy to meet with you . . ."

He suggested they meet at Alice's on the Malibu pier. "Is this evening too soon?"

"If you don't mind me coming in my jogging outfit . . . tonight's my regular spa time . . ."

"Fine with me."

Now, seated overlooking the old railroad pier, considered to be an historic landmark, they were munching on hard French rolls awaiting their dinner. No wonder Anne fell in love with him, she mused. He had dressed casually in jeans and turtleneck, topped with a light blazer. He looks too thin and tired, she observed, but understandable under the circumstances.

"Please call me Ben," he began. "And, may I call you Carolyn?" She appeared not to notice the admiring glances she had attracted as they were being seated. Indeed, dressed as she was, in her designer, aqua jogging suit, the young woman's shoulder-length platinum blonde hair would catch anyone's eye.

"Please do . . ."

He hadn't dined with a woman since Anne's death and found it difficult to suppress the twinge of disloyalty. Focused on the morbidity of his project, as he had been, Carolyn's obvious enjoyment with life in general was a pleasant relief.

He found it difficult to break the ice, so she took the initiative. "Thanks for the invitation . . . in such nice surroundings," she smiled. "Now, how can I help you?"

"How well did you know my wife?"

"Rather well, I think. We frequently had lunch together. We shared some of our healing and health philosophies . . ."

Ben raised his eyebrows. "Oh . . . healing and health philosophies? What do you mean?"

She regarded him levelly. "Before I answer that question, Ben, allow me to ask you: how well did you know how your wife actually felt about her profession?"

The question caught him off guard. "Quite well, I thought."

"Thought?"

"Well, yes. We talked quite a bit. And I thought I knew her feelings quite well. But, now that I've read her Journal . . ." He spread his hands in a gesture of wonder. "Now, I *really* know how she thought. I wish I'd known then what I know now . . ."

Carolyn again took the initiative. "Did the two of you ever talk about, or discuss, different modalities . . ."

"Are you referring to alternative medicine?"

"Yes, that's what I mean," she responded.

"We did some. Especially when her grandmother was so ill. With lymphoma. She talked then about laetrile. Her grandparents had asked her about it."

Carolyn was absently tracing a design on the tablecloth. "Did she do any personal research on the subject?"

"More than I realized at the time."

Suddenly Carolyn changed her tack. "How well did you know Dr. Rush's father?"

"Bertram Collins? Not well. I met him a couple of times. Once before our wedding. Then, of course, at the wedding. Actually, I don't personally know him very well. Mostly I knew him through Anne. Why do you ask?"

"Before I answer that question, let me ask another. Do you know how Collins felt about alternative modalities . . . in particular those that treat patients with few or no drugs?"

Ben furrowed his brow in concentration. "No . . . I guess I don't know how he felt. Why, do you know something that I don't know?"

Carolyn eyed Ben contemplatively over her glass as she took a sip of water. "I might. I just might. I'm not sure. But let me ask one more question . . . okay?"

He shrugged. "Of course. I don't know where you're going. But, shoot."

"When was the last time Dr. Rush saw her father?"

"Why, when we were in San Francisco . . . to attend her grandfather's funeral."

"Were you with her at that meeting?" Carolyn asked.

"No. I took her, then left her. And picked her up later."

Carolyn took a deep breath. "Do you know what transpired at that meeting? What they talked about?"

"Not really. Anne was quite upset after the meeting. But that was nothing unusual. She was always upset when she met — or talked with — her father . . ."

Neither spoke for a couple of minutes, but concentrated on their dinner. Suddenly Ben dropped his fork. "Look, Carolyn, I've got the idea that you know something I should know. Do you?"

She laughed. "Ben, I like you. I don't know what I expected. But, you're direct. I like that."

She adopted a sober mien. "Ben, I don't like thinking the things I am thinking. But the thought has nagged me, ever since you and Dr. Rush returned from San Francisco that time . . ."

Ben noticed how pale she had suddenly become. "What thought, Carolyn? What do you mean?"

She was pushing a piece of fish around with her fork. "I'm not sure. But some pieces are beginning to come together . . . pieces that didn't make sense before . . ."

"What kind of pieces?" he urged.

She looked up. "Ben, forgive me if I am wrong. I hope I am. But the idea's stuck in my head . . . the idea that Dr. Rush's father — Bertram Collins — had more to do with his daughter's death than we realize . . ."

CHAPTER NINETEEN

Ben's mind was in a whirl. The possibility that Collins — Anne's own father — could have been directly or indirectly implicated in his daughter's demise, as Carolyn suggested, was inconceivable. But, given the nature of the man as he knew him, the more Ben thought about it, *almost* inconceivable seemed a more accurate term.

However, when it came right down to it, Carolyn's suspicions were just that: suspicions. Which she admitted.

The next step was to talk to Allen Drury. Except for the fact that he had been Anne's employer, Ben doubted that time spent with the doctor would add much to his fund of knowledge. Realizing that Ben was an investigative journalist, and wondering why he should suddenly show up two years after Anne's death, Drury warily suggested they meet at his office at six.

Because it was traffic rush hour, Ben allowed himself plenty of time. He parked in the underground garage and took the elevator. It was precisely six o'clock when he entered the tastefully-decorated waiting room.

Carolyn was gathering her things in preparation for leaving. She smiled. "Thanks again for the dinner." She indicated Drury's office down the hall. "I just talked to Dr. Drury. He told me to tell you he'll be with you in about five minutes. See you."

Then she was gone, leaving behind her an aura of life and joy. Suddenly Ben realized how much he had enjoyed their time together last night.

Ben looked around. The decor was well done and bore what he judged to be a woman's touch. Carolyn's? He doubted it. Probably a professional decorator. He heard a door open and looked up in time to see Drury approaching him. He had shed his white coat and wore an expensive, camel-hair sport coat.

His first impressions of the man were: overweight, with a lack-of-sunshine pallor and calculating eyes. But the man's single, most outstanding feature were his ears. They were the most prominent ears Ben had ever seen on a man, although they were partially covered by long, but well-styled hair.

Drury's hand was extended in greeting. "Ben, it's good to meet you. I suppose we should have met before. But . . . that's the way it is with busy people . . ."

He motioned in the direction of the hallway. "Come, let's go into my office. More comfortable than here . . ."

The office also bore the same earmarks of opulence as the rest of the complex. "May I offer you a drink? Or coffee?"

Ben declined.

"It's been a long day. I'll have a little relaxer . . ." He poured himself a generous glass of Scotch and pulled up a chair.

"Well," he began, "nice of you to come all this way to meet me here. Sorry to request it, but I've got a meeting here in Beverly Hills shortly . . ."

"Perfectly all right," Ben said. "I've been in town all day anyway. No problem to drop over here."

Drury extracted a small bottle from his vest pocket and shook a couple of yellow capsules in his hand. Downing them with a swallow of the liquor, he explained. "Touch of high blood pressure . . . probably should find a good doctor."

Chuckling at his own joke, Drury said, "Ben, you've no idea how distressing it's been without Anne. She was one of the finest clinicians I've ever worked with . . . besides that, she was a wonderful woman. We miss her . . ."

"So do I," Ben answered. "Thanks for the good words . . ."

Drury drained the glass and set it down. "I suspect this isn't just a social call, Ben. What can I do for you?"

Ben said, "I see that you graduated from Stanford . . ."

"Yes. Wonderful school. San Francisco's my home. It was just natural that I'd choose Stanford . . ."

San Francisco, Ben thought. Carolyn said Drury and Collins had been talking on the telephone the day that Anne was in the hospital. Mere coincidence?

Aloud, he asked, "Did you and Anne ever discuss her illness? Her lymphoma?"

"Yes. But not at length. I suggested she see Dr. Cranston. Excellent surgeon. You know Cranston? Yes, of course you do. Why do you ask?"

"Well, I've been reading Anne's journal . . ." Purposely, he watched for a reaction from Drury. He was not disappointed. The man's pallor dropped another shade. "You knew, of course, that Anne kept a journal?"

Drury rose and walked to the window. By the time he turned, he had managed to compose himself. "Journal? No, not really. What kind of a journal?"

"She kept record of just about everything having to do with her professional life. Her career. Some personal things as well. But mostly professional. She started it at Stanford when one of

her professors suggested it. Kept it up till the day
. . . till a few days before she died . . ."

Ben noticed Drury's hands trembling. Almost
without thinking the man downed another couple of
yellow capsules. "Anyway," he went on, "I was
reading where Anne mentioned something about
seeking what she called 'alternative therapy' for her
lymphoma."

By now Drury was in control. "Well, of course
we discussed alternative therapies. That's mostly
quack medicine, you know. But I strongly advised she
take the tried and true route . . ."

"You mean surgery?" Ben asked casually.

"Yes. Surgery and chemo. That's chemotherapy.
And radiation. These are *proven* therapies." Drury's
voice was stronger now that he was on familiar
territory.

"Did the two of your ever discuss laetrile?"

Drury cocked his head as though thinking.
"Laetrile. We may have, but I rather doubt it. The
stuff was really controversial during the 70s, but it's
sort of faded out now . . ."

Ben opened his attache case and pulled out a
sheaf of notes. "Anne was saying something about a
Dr. Richardson. Berkeley man, I believe. Said she
talked with him. Did she share any of that
conversation with you?"

Drury was quite evidently becoming nervous.
"Richardson. Oh, yes. Advocate of laetrile, as I recall.
Yes, Anne did mention the man's name. I suggested
she keep away from him . . . he was under fire . . .
by the American Medical Association. And for her to
have her name linked with Richardson . . ."

"Not good professionally?" Ben said softly.

"Yes. Yes, that's exactly what I told her. Yes, I
remember it all rather clearly now." Beads of sweat
were running down his face and he ran a finger
around the inside of his collar.

Chapter Nineteen

He glanced at his watch. "I didn't know it was so late. Ben, it's been good, but I've really . . ."

Ben slid the papers back into his attache case and closed it. He arose and stuck out his hand. "I understand, Allen. Thanks a lot for your time. Another time, maybe?"

"Sure. Maybe we can do lunch or dinner."

They started walking down the hallway. Suddenly Ben stopped. "Oh, Allen, the thought just came. Do you by any chance happen to know Bertram Collins, Anne's father?"

Drury step wavered and his mouth dropped open. "Uh . . . Collins, you say? Anne's father. Uh . . ."

Ben appeared not to notice the man's discomfiture. "Yes, the prominent San Francisco attorney. You must have heard of him. And, since you both come from the same city, I thought . . ."

The shrilling telephone interrupted them. Relief written all over his face, Drury hurried over to Carolyn's desk and picked up the instrument.

"Hello . . . uh, oh, I was about to leave. Uh, I can't talk right now. Uh, sure, sure, I'll call you back."

When Drury hung up the telephone and faced Ben, he looked like he might faint. "Sorry," he said, "but, I've got to leave. Emergency. You understand."

Ben grinned. "I understand. Thanks again for the time. You've been more helpful than you know . . ."

As soon as he let Ben out the door, Drury scuttled to his office and dialed Collins' number. "Bert, I *couldn't* talk right then. Ben Rush was here. Ben Rush, your son-in-law. What was he doing? He was asking a lot of questions . . .!"

Ben dialed Carolyn's number. She answered immediately. "Hi, I told you I'd call afterwards . . ."

"How did it go?" she asked. "I've been on pins and needles wondering . . ."

"Depends how you mean it. If you're wondering about just the meeting, it went fine."

"I mean, did you learn anything? About . . ."

"Drury and Collins? I think so. I'm quite sure of it. The man was nervous as a cat." He drew a long breath. "Carolyn, I don't want to put you in a difficult position by all of this."

"I know, Ben. I know. Dr. Rush was such a fine person . . . and I just want to do what I can . . ."

"There is something."

"What?"

"I think it's time for me to meet Jack Drury. And if it's not too much trouble, I'd like for you to introduce us . . ."

Laetrile, Ben thought, where better to get started than with laetrile. What is the stuff? Where does it come from? Why is there so much controversy over laetrile? He checked Anne's books. No mention of laetrile in the *Merck Manual*, nor in the *PDR*, the *Physician's Desk Reference*. He struck out in *Mosby's Medical and Nursing Dictionary*. Finally, in *Dorland's Medical Dictionary, 27th Edition*, after the statement that laetrile "is alleged to have antineoplastic properties," Ben found the statement that laetrile was "sometimes used interchangeably with *amygdalin*."

Under *amygdalin* in *Dorland's*, he read, "A cyanogenetic glycoside (followed by its lengthy chemical description) . . . characteristically found in seeds and other plant parts of members of the Rosaceae family, i.e., *almonds*"[21]

Now, Ben thought, I might be getting somewhere. He looked up the word *antineoplastic*, a term described as having the ability to check "the maturation and proliferation of malignant cells." [22]

Chapter Nineteen

"In other words," Ben said aloud in amazement, "laetrile isn't a drug. It's a natural substance . . . one that apparently does have at least *some* ability to inhibit cancer cells. And if that's indeed the case, why all the fuss and fury?"

A telephone call from Ross Hannibal was soon to give Ben the answer to that question with all its ramifications. "I've got some valuable information on laetrile for you," Hannibal said. "Some things I think you should have before you get too deeply involved in your research. . ."

"Oh . . . I was just on my way to the cabin for the weekend," Ben said. "Why don't you join me there for dinner?"

"What're you serving?"

"I make the freshest salad in Malibu . . . and broil a great salmon fillet. How about it?"

"Tell me how to get there . . ."

Lyman Prescott, until the mid-70s, had been a respected and respectable family physician, who lived and practiced in Alameda, California. Conservative in every way, no one would have foreseen that Dr. Prescott was to become embroiled in one of the hottest, most-bitterly fought medical controversies of the century.

Thin almost to a fault, with a prominent Adam's apple that bobbed up and down as he talked, Prescott appeared almost to be a comic strip character. Because he wore a suit at least two sizes too large for him, that flapped in the breeze as he strode briskly down the street or a hospital hall, some of his friends lovingly referred to him as Ichabod Crane.

The man's physical appearance belied his competence and his dedication to his profession. In the entire Oakland/Alameda area, he was probably the last remaining family doctor who made house calls. Which made him busier than the busiest.

Dr. Anne's Journal

He was happy going about his business trying to help keep people well.

But he was deeply troubled by the fact that he, along with most other physicians that he knew, were unsuccessful in their treatment of patients with cancer. He didn't include all doctors in that categorization, because there was *one* doctor he knew who was becoming quite famous for his success in that area. That man was Dr. John A. Richardson[23], who, like Prescott, had practiced medicine in the East Bay area for over twenty years.

The two had known each other for most of those years. Due to the heavy patient load each man carried, they seldom saw each other personally as they had when their practices were smaller. They did, however, confer frequently by telephone.

Across the years, both men faithfully prescribed all of the currently accepted modalities for cancer treatment: surgery, radiation and chemotherapy, most of which they referred to specialists in those fields. Individually, and without discussing the matter with each other, the two men noted that such therapies seldom prolonged the lives of their patients . . .

In fact, as Lyman protested bitterly to his wife one day, "All that we're doing for cancer patients seems to be eroding the quality of their lives, and then hastening their death . . ."

"But, Lyman, you're doing the best that you know," she said.

"That's true, but it's not enough."

"What do you mean?"

"Because, in view of the expense to the patient — who is already suffering the tortures of the damned — it looks like we're just adding to his problems. Instead of easing his pain, we're heaping on the side effects of radiation burns and drug toxicity . . ."

"But, Lyman, what can you do?"

Chapter Nineteen

"I don't know. But I've got to do something . . ."

Prescott first heard of laetrile from one of his cancer patients.

"Doc, why don't you treat me with the same stuff that Dr. Richardson is using," the woman asked.

"Oh, what *is* Dr. Richardson using that I'm not?"

"He calls it Laetrile. And it works. Ask him about it."

When he got home from his house calls that evening, Prescott telephoned his friend and asked him about "Laetrile," the "new cancer therapy" he was using with such good results. Richardson invited him to, "Come over take a look."

The next morning when Lyman Prescott visited Richardson's office in Berkeley, both his practice and his life were changed forever. Following Richardson's advice, Prescott "went right to the source" and contacted Dr. Ernst T. Krebs, Sr. and his sons, who lived in San Francisco. Not only had Krebs and his two sons developed Laetrile, but they had been working with it in the Bay area for almost fifty years[24].

Soon, as Richardson had done, Prescott began utilizing Laetrile in his practice, with the same results: His patients began reporting a reduction in pain, increased appetites and a gradual return of strength. In addition, almost miraculously, their mental outlooks improved[25].

Hannibal shoved back his plate and folded his napkin. *"That . . ."* he said, *"was* a great meal. Excellent, in fact."

"No problem. My specialty . . . along with baked potatoes and the fixin's . . ."

"Well, as I was saying . . . things were going well for Prescott and Richardson, all of them . . . then all hell broke loose!"

"What do you mean?"

"They were raided . . . and shut down."

Ben was incredulous. "Shut down? On what charges?"

"That's a long story. I suggest you ask Prescott himself."

"How can I do that?"

Hannibal grinned. "The same way I got the information I just gave you — up in Alameda . . ."

"You mean . . .?"

"That's right. I heard about Prescott, decided to do some digging, and flew up there yesterday. Want to know more?"

"*Absolutely*! This kind of information's vital."

"That's what I thought," Hannibal said. He fumbled in his shirt pocket and pulled out a square of paper. "Here's Prescott's card." Ben accepted it with a thrill of anticipation.

Now, seated in Dr. Lyman Prescott's tiny, but very neat living room on Central Avenue in Alameda, he was listening to the man's story.

"For a couple of years," Prescott said sadly, "I was happy, perhaps the happiest I'd ever been as a doctor. After treating them with laetrile, my patients were eating better. They were feeling better, even looking better . . ."

"Then what happened?" Ben asked.

"The Feds came in and took it all away," Prescott said. He looked tired, Ben thought. Depressed and wornout. And ancient. He was also terribly thin, which emphasized the old man's prominent Adam's apple that bobbed up and down as he talked. Ben noticed that Prescott also had the nervous habit of wringing his hands together as he talked.

"But I don't understand how they could do that," Ben said. "At that time laetrile was legal, wasn't it?"

"We thought so . . . Richardson and I. The
Krebs thought so. But, then, poof! just like that, they
swooped in . . ."

"And that was the beginning of trouble?"

The old doctor nodded. "Right. That was the
beginning. At the time we didn't know it, but it really
was . . ."

Ben had telephoned Lyman Prescott the
morning following his meeting with Hannibal, and
explained his interest in the subject. It seemed that
Prescott was eager to talk to anybody seeking the
facts. So, Ben had flown to the Bay area that same
afternoon. He had rented a car and driven to
Alameda.

From the look on Prescott's face, he appeared
to be a man who had suffered a great deal. Probably
as much as any of his patients, Ben thought.

"I appreciate having this opportunity of talking
with you," Ben said, "because it's obvious you're well-
acquainted with the subject of laetrile . . ."

Prescott acknowledged the statement with a
nod.

"Mr. Hannibal gave me the background of your
story. So, now, if you don't mind, I'd like you to tell
me exactly what laetrile is, and how it works. Will
you do that?"

"Sure. Be glad to . . ."

Laetrile, Prescott told Ben, is a glycoside, a
type of carbohydrate. It is found all over the globe,
occurring naturally in about 1,200 different plants.
"In fact," Prescott said, "laetrile, also called Vitamin
B-17, is so common that everybody has taken laetrile
many times . . ."

"That's hard to believe."

"I know," Prescott said, "but it's true. A few of
the plants laetrile is found in are chick peas and
lentils, lima beans and Chinese sprouts, cashews and

alfalfa, barley, brown rice . . . just to name a few
. . ."

"How about apricot seeds?"

Prescott nodded. "Yes, apricot seeds as well.
For commercial purposes, laetrile is derived from the
kernels of the apricot, the peach and the bitter
almond . . ."

"I suppose, then, that laetrile is of fairly new
or recent, origin, isn't it?"

"Oh, no. Laetrile's use in medicine was well-
known among Chinese, Egyptians and Arab
physicians thousands of years ago."[26]

Ben was puzzled. "Then I don't understand
what's behind all the problems surrounding laetrile."

For the first time, Prescott smiled. "I'm still
trying to understand . . ."

"Anyway, you got involved with laetrile shortly
after Dr. John Richardson got involved. Right?"

"Right."

"Now, for the big question, the one I suspect
being asked by everybody: *How* does laetrile work on
cancer?"

"Before I answer that question," Prescott said,
"I've got to tell you this — no matter what you may
have heard, nobody ever said that laetrile would cure
cancer. Nothing cures cancer. Only the body itself,
when it's given the right environment, can cure
cancer."

"Okay," Ben agreed, "I understand."

"Well, then, basically, here's the theory behind
the use of laetrile in cancer therapy . . ."

Step by step, in very logical fashion, Prescott
walked Ben through his research. "Cancer," he said,
"is a chronic metabolic disease. It is chronic in that
it's a disease of long standing that cannot heal itself
. . ."

"I get it," Ben interjected, "and it's metabolic
because it originates in the body and is in some way

involved with the digestion and the assimilation of food . . ."

"Exactly," Prescott said, "and since cancer cannot be transmitted to a healthy person, it is, as I said, a chronic, metabolic disease. That means, that if cancer is in someway associated with *metabolism*, that a nutrient, or nutrients, are missing from the diet to make people sick. This theory, by the way, is being consistently proven to be correct."

"Does that mean," Ben asked with some excitement, "that if that or those missing nutrients are restored to the diet, then the body should respond and get well? Is that right?"

Prescott nodded. "Well . . . yes . . . basically, that's right. But, before we get too far afield, let me explain how laetrile works . . ."

Prescott explained the theory as Richardson understood it, which was the basis for his extensive work. Cancer, Richardson had said, was not some strange invading force from outside the body. Rather, it was a malfunction of normal mechanisms solely within the body itself.

Those malfunctions, Richardson had theorized, were the result of a deficiency in a chemical substance found in certain foods, in addition to a deficiency in the pancreatic enzymes known as the trypsins.

The deficiency in the chemical food substance, Prescott told Ben, is a cyanide-containing compound, called amygdalin or B-17.

"Otherwise known as *laetrile*!" Ben added.

"Exactly," Prescott said. "But, there is more. And this is one of the primary functions of laetrile. Laetrile will only release its cyanide in the presence of an enzyme group called glucuronidase, which is to be found in appreciable amounts *only in cancer tissue*."

Ben digested that for a moment before he asked, "Then, what's the bottom line?"

"The bottom line, as you call it, or the net result, is that cancer cells are unable to withstand the cyanide in the laetrile, or B-17, *and are destroyed.*"

"What about the normal, non-cancerous cells? How do they respond to laetrile?"

"That's the second primary function of laetrile. The normal, non-cancerous cells are not threatened by the cyanide. In fact, they are able to convert that cyanide into nutritional substances that are vital to one's health . . ."

Prescott paused, "But there is a catch."

"What's that?"

"Unless we eat the foods that contain this very necessary vitamin, then our bodies' miraculous mechanisms won't produce the miracle of healing we are seeking . . ."

Both men were quiet after this announcement.

Then Ben asked slowly, "But you said that laetrile, or B-17, is found in hundreds of foods. Right?"

"Right. But, Ben, when our diets consist more and more of devitalized, highly-processed foods, filled with chemicals and additives . . . then, the nutrients we need — including the cancer-fighting forces of laetrile — are refined out of our food. And, we are left naked and without defense . . ."

CHAPTER TWENTY

Laetrile. Ben was finding himself completely sensitized to the subject. Thoughts on the controversial substance seemed to permeate the very air that he breathed. At the same time he was suddenly aware of a paradox: Anne had recorded very little about laetrile in her Journal. Why? he asked himself.

She had not been unaware of the substance. He knew that for a fact, because on a few occasions he remembered that she had spoken of the use of laetrile in the treatment of cancer. At the time he had shown little interest and the subject was dropped. Now, realizing his wife's non-aggressive nature, Ben spent hours in self flagellation.

If only I had known her situation, he groaned. If only I had listened more carefully to her spoken and *unspoken* words. If only, if only . . . he berated himself, till his guilt paralyzed his thinking processes and his work ground to a halt.

He shared his torment with Carolyn. She listened to his recriminations for part of one evening, then abruptly arose from the table and slipped on her jacket.

"Goodnight, Ben," she said and slid her chair back.

Startled, he asked, "Where are you going?"

"Home . . ."

He checked his watch. "But . . . it's early . . ."

"Yes, it is early . . ."

"But, tomorrow's Sunday . . . and . . ."

"I know all of that, Ben. But, I've got more to do than to listen to you flog yourself over something you couldn't have helped at the time. Nor can you do anything about it now . . ."

Stunned at her directness, he stammered, "But . . . I . . . I should have known. Should have been able to help her . . . but I didn't. So I failed her. Can't you see that?"

Unexpectedly she laughed. "Ben . . . Ben. Anne loved you. And you loved her. Can't you remember that? And forget the other? You did all you could have done. And your lives were good . . . now it's time to move on. You're still young. Act like it."

Speechlessly, he let her go.

The moment he returned to his condo, he dialed her number. "I want to apologize . . ." he began.

She laughed ntly. "Ben. No need. Just remember, you *didn't* fail Anne. Not in any way. But you *could* fail her now . . . and you *will*, unless you become unparalyzed and get to work."

He digested that a moment then said soberly. "Carolyn, you really shook me tonight when you walked out. You gave me the jolt I needed. You woke me up. Now, I'm back on the job again."

"Good . . . now, goodnight."

"Wait, Carolyn. Wait. May I call you again?"

"Yes," she said softly. "With a progress report. Then we'll consider taking it from there. Goodnight, Ben."

"You're right, of course. Thank you. Goodnight, Carolyn."

Ben shook himself as though awakening from a deep sleep and slid a yellow pad from his brief case. Across the top he wrote: "Anne and Laetrile." Then he racked his memory to recall those few instances when she had mentioned laetrile. In general, he remembered that the subject had come up. But that was all.

He opened the photocopy of Anne's journal and began leafing through it, searching for references to the substance . . .

It was slow going. Often Anne had taken her time to write, and had carefully penned every word. Other times, when hurried or tired, her hand took on the stereotypical "prescription scribble" of many doctors.

Not until her second year in med school did she mention laetrile, then only in passing . . .

> *Professor Jacobs suggested that we don't even think about what he called 'unproven modalities.' He said, 'You've got enough to think about that is legitimate.' When someone asked what he meant, Jacobs said, 'Laetrile is unproven. Till it has been accepted by the FDA, forget it. Leave it alone. Don't even waste time reading or thinking about it.'. . .*

Ben noted the date and flipped more pages. Month after month, with nothing, then . . .

> *Guest lecturer from the FDA today in Pharmacology 420. He seemed quite knowledgeable. He spoke about the process of licensing new drugs. In the process he strongly denounced doctors who treat patients with laetrile and 'other untested drugs' such as 'laetrile.' When a student asked if laetrile had ever been licensed, the answer was, 'No. Attempts have been made by laetrilists to secure an IND (Investigational New*

*Drug license), but to date such efforts
have not been successful'. . .*[27]

By now it was getting late. Ben had brewed himself
a cup of herbal tea then went back at it. Aside from
those two brief notes, there were no other entries
regarding laetrile until after she had finished med
school, married, completed her internship and had
begun private practice.

His eyes were tired and he was about ready to
quit for the night, when, among Anne's notes
concerning her grandmother's illness, he found this
entry:

*November 21 — Grandfather and
Grandmother asked me if I knew
anything about laetrile. At that moment
I knew that my blessed grandmother
was dying. She and Grandfather were
reaching out to me for help. And I had
no help to give them. Of course I knew
what laetrile was. Or at least I thought
I did. All I could tell them was what I
had been told, i.e., that it 'hadn't been
properly tested.' Even as I told them
that, I wasn't certain if that was
actually the truth, because I had never
attempted to find out more on the
subject for myself. God help them. God
help me. I desperately want to help my
Grandmother. But, I don't know how
. . .*

Now it was coming clear to him. When she
returned from San Francisco that time, Anne *had*
spoken about laetrile.

"What good is a doctor who can't help her
loved ones?" she asked miserably.

"But you are helping them. Your love and your
. . ."

"Ben, that's not what I mean. Grandmother is
sick. Really sick. They asked me for my opinion.
Their doctor is suggesting surgery. And after that,
chemotherapy and radiation . . ."

"What else is there?"

"They asked me about laetrile . . ."

"Laetrile. I've heard the word," Ben said. "But,
that's about it . . ."

"I don't know much more, Ben. Except, here
and there, I have heard that it has been successfully
used in cancer therapy . . ."

Ben was amazed. "Then . . . why don't you tell
them that?"

"Because . . ." she started, then suddenly burst
into tears. "Oh, Ben, Grandmother is dying of cancer.
Of *cancer*. And . . . I . . . I'm a doctor. And . . . *I
can't help her*! . . ."

Her Journal open before him now, Ben relived
that scene. Anne had cried herself to sleep. Then,
during the night when he awoke to go to the
bathroom, he realized she was not in bed — and her
side of the bed was cold.

He had found her kneeling beside the sofa in
the living room. Weeping and praying. He knelt
beside her and put his arm around her shoulders.
After a while she allowed him to lead her back to
bed. Neither one of them slept much after that . . .

Immediately following this Journal entry, Ben
noticed what he had not seen before: Anne's search
. . .

*December 10 — Ben must be right when
he said, "the majority of cancer cure
researchers are spinning their wheels
and are looking in the wrong places." I
feel so helpless when patients come to*

*me with their illness, their diseases. Yes,
and their cancer. I'm not God, though
we were trained to almost believe that as
medical doctors we are. There must be a
way — or ways — to reverse the terrible
destructive force of cancer.*

And again . . .

*February 5 — Grandmother is dying.
She knows it. Grandfather knows it.
And I know it. She is so loving, so
beautiful, so needed by the world. And I
am helpless to do anything for her,
except stand by and watch her waste
away.*

Then, that black day that he remembered so
clearly . . .

*April 11 — She is gone now. My beloved
Grandmother is gone. What is left of her
brutalized body is in the grave. There
must be a way to prevent such horrible,
such torturous, useless cachexia. Such
untimely deaths. Would God that I could
be used as an instrument in finding that
way.*

His voice tight with righteous anger, Ben
whispered hoarsely, "Dear Anne, I promise you that
you will not have died in vain. And that your prayers
will be realized: that you — even beyond the grave —
will be an instrument of healing, an instrument to
prevent the uselessness of the cancer decimation we
now see. With God as my witness, I swear it . . ."
Ben's back and shoulders ached. But he could
not stop where he was. Putting on a light sweater, he
stepped out into the night. High in the heavens he

studied some of the constellations he remembered
from his months at sea . . .

Orion, the Hunter. Cassiopeia's Chair. The Big
Dipper. As he had done so often, Ben followed the
two pointer stars and found the Polar Star. The
North Star, used by countless thousands of seamen to
guide them to their safe harbor. Many a long night
on bow watch, he had watched as the Dipper pivoted
around that star.

Ah, and there was Venus, the Evening Star
. . .

What was it Anne had whispered that night?
Yes, those words from Tennyson — "Sunset and
evening star, and one clear call for me. And may
there by no moaning at the bar, when I put out to
sea."

May there be no moaning at the bar . . .

It was then that her presence surrounded him
like a cloud, a bright, almost tangible aura. And Ben
knew — as Anne had promised — that her spirit was
guiding him.

. . . no moaning at the bar . . .

He pulled his sweater more tightly around his
shoulders. A cool, brisk breezed caressed his face,
then was gone. And with it, the aura that he had
more felt than seen. He felt refreshed. Now he would
go back to work.

From that point in her Journal, Anne had
seemed obsessed with cancer. She saw it in the clinic.
She read it in the medical journals. She wrote . . .
she struggled . . . she sought ways and means to
defeat it. But, in the end, it defeated her . . .

Fingers trembling, Ben turned to the page he
most dreaded to read. But this time he read it with
anticipation: because he *knew* she had written an
underlying message just for him. A message that he
alone would comprehend.

"How will I know how to use your Journal?"
he had asked.

Dr. Anne's Journal

"You will know, Ben, you *will* know . . ."

October 19 — Today, I know as fact
what I have long suspected and can no
longer hide it from myself. I have
cancer. Lymphoma. I know my intuitive
diagnosis will be confirmed objectively.
But, from this day, I will live each day
more fully. I will seek more diligently
for ways to free others from this scourge.

Scribbled in the margin of that page was a brief note, penned with a different instrument. "Ben, I hope your skills succeed where mine have failed . . ."

CHAPTER TWENTY-ONE

Marina Del Rey was Ben's favorite marina, one that he and Anne had frequently visited to traverse the waterfront and watch the boats. This Sunday afternoon, though, the purpose of his visit to the marina was for business. Following Carolyn's directions, he parked in the underground garage of her condo and took the elevator to the tenth floor.

She opened the door immediately.

He caught his breath. Outlined momentarily against the floor-to-ceiling window, with her healthy tan and blonde hair, Carolyn was stunning. "Come in . . . come in," she said. "We're waiting . . ."

As he stepped inside and she guided him into the living room with its unsurpassed overview of the marina, he became aware of the other person.

"Ben," she was saying, "meet Jack Drury. Jack, this is Ben Rush . . ."

The man was tall, lithe, athletic looking, and well-tanned. His grip was firm, his gaze steady, his smile warm. Yet, without a word spoken, each man instantly recognized the other as a competitor. That unbidden awareness startled Ben. Not until this moment had he fostered any proprietary notions toward Carolyn.

"Carolyn has told me much about you," Jack was saying as they seated themselves. "And I understand you're digging into an area that I'm very much interested in."

Ben nodded, wondering exactly what Carolyn had said.

"Yes," he spoke aloud, "Carolyn did indicate that you've done considerable research into alternative therapies . . ."

If Carolyn was aware of the propriety interest the men sensed, she ignored it, quietly moving about serving them hors d'oeuvres and tall glasses of lemonade.

When she had served them and seated herself, Carolyn joined them. "It seems," she began, "that the two of you are on such parallel courses, though for different reasons, that I thought you should meet . . . to share ideas, compare notes, whatever."

Ben nodded. "Thanks, Carolyn." Then he addressed Jack. "I met your father a few days ago . . ."

Jack chuckled easily. "How did your meeting go?"

"What do you mean?"

"Well, my father's adamantly opposed to anything that smacks of anything having to do with what he calls 'those quacks' . . . and if he had any idea where you were going . . . who knows what he might say . . ." He shrugged. "So, depending, it could have been rough going. Was it?"

Ben waggled his hand. "Let's say it was interesting." He was feeling his way, not really knowing what to expect. How much did Jack know, he wondered, and exactly where was he coming from?

An impasse. Obviously at this point neither man wanted to commit himself positionally. Carolyn broke the ice.

"Ben, didn't you say that Dr. Drury seemed quite nervous?"

Might as well take the plunge, Ben thought. "Yes. In fact, I'd say he was *quite* nervous . . ." He surveyed Jack's reaction, but there was none.

He went on, "So nervous that he . . ." He paused. "Jack, did you know your father had high blood pressure?"

"High blood pressure? No, he doesn't. I mean, not that I knew of. Why?"

"Well, as soon as I got there he offered me a drink. Which I declined. He said he'd had a rough day, so he poured himself a shot of Scotch . . ."

Jack was leaning back, arms across his chest, a noncommittal expression on his face.

"Then," Ben went on, "a couple of times while I was there, he swallowed a couple of yellow capsules . . ."

Jack paled. "*Yellow* capsules? Are you sure?"

"Certain. The first time he said something about his high blood pressure. Joked something about needing a good doctor. The second time he seemed not to be aware of taking the capsules. Sort of reflex action . . ."

Jack looked troubled. "I had no idea."

Ben shrugged. "Anyway, I asked him about Anne . . . about their discussions concerning her cancer . . ."

"And?" Jack picked up when Ben paused.

"He told me that he had strongly recommended that Anne follow the traditional route . . ."

"I know that route." Ben noticed the tinge of cynicism as Jack spoke the words.

"I brought up the subject of the Berkeley doctor, man by the name of John Richardson . . . and his work with laetrile . . ."

"Richardson?" Jack raised his eyebrows. "Don't know the man. How did Dad react?"

"Seemed to get more nervous. That was when he came on strong about laetrile. Assured me that he'd strongly insisted Anne keep away from Richardson's people. That all of them were under fire by the AMA. Insisted it wouldn't have been good for her to have her name linked with any of them . . ."

Jack laughed bitterly. "I know what you're talking about."

"Then," Ben said, watching Jack narrowly, "I asked him if he knew Bertram Collins, my late wife's father . . ."

Jack's expression didn't change. "I've never met the man. But Dad did. Spoke of him frequently. They'd grown up in the same area. Suburb of San Francisco. Went to Stanford together . . ."

Until this moment Carolyn had been a bystander. But at this revelation, she burst out, "Stanford!" Then put her hand over her mouth in embarrassment.

Both men looked at her questioningly.

"I'm sorry to speak out like that," she apologized. "Now it's coming together . . ."

"What's coming together?" Ben asked.

"Those phone calls. They *must* have been Mr. Collins. He would call, refused to give his name, but demand to speak to Dr. Drury. He was very rude on the telephone . . ."

"Did he call often?" Jack asked.

"Fairly often . . . but it seems like he called more often *after* you left the practice. And . . . now it's beginning to make sense . . . every time the man called, your father, Jack, was always very upset and nervous the rest of the day . . ."

"I wonder why?" Ben asked. "I wonder why . . ."

Jory Ralston rarely came to his office on Sundays, but had made an exception this time. As an employee of the Federal Drug Administration, he knew he was not to have been targeted for political or personal pressures from outside the FDA. And, for the most part, he was not. However, the situation he was now facing was unlike anything he had ever known . . .

Chapter Twenty-One

For more than a dozen years after receiving his medical degree from Columbia, Ralston had practiced medicine in Waverly, a bedroom community composed mainly of lower-ranking military officers from the Pentagon. As commuting goes, the forty-mile drive to the center of Washington, D.C. wasn't excessive, and most of Waverly's commuters carpooled.

Jory Ralston and his young bride had fit in well in the community and began making plans to remain there indefinitely. Then something went wrong, something that changed the course of his life forever. The guilty secret locked within his breast, Jory packed a single suitcase and drove to the capitol, where he spent the night in a motel. The next morning he followed up on the suggestion of a former patient and applied for a position at the Federal Drug Administration.

The only position open for a physician was processing NDAs, New Drug Applications. From what little he knew about the FDA, coupled with what he learned from the initial interview, he realized the task would be tedious, endless, probably boring, and he would be eternally buried in an avalanche of paper.

After what had transpired, all Jory Ralston wanted was to be buried, in paper or otherwise, for the rest of his natural life, however long that might be. Hopefully, then, he could forget the tragedy that had sucked the life out of him.

As fate would have it, Ralston's first assignment was to process the NDA for Oncoplex, a new cancer drug developed by BII, Bullion, Inc., International. A month before Ralston accepted the position with the FDA, BII had delivered its NDA for Oncoplex on a truck. A truck had been necessary, because the Oncoplex NDA consisted of over 100,000 printed pages, 283 volumes in all.

Dr. Anne's Journal

For more than one month the entire consignment — which was required by law, and which covered more than two years of testing on animals and humans — had set in the cubbyhole of an office, which Ralston inherited. The material jammed the tiny, airless room, leaving barely enough floor space for Ralston, a desk and a filing cabinet.

Now, nearly two months into the project, Ralston had barely made a dent in the massive stack of technical data that was his responsibility to read, evaluate and pass on.

Not that it mattered to him. Hidden from public view, he literally buried himself in his work. Time meant nothing to him. He had nowhere to go and nothing to do. He was merely existing, which was his total future as far as he could visualize it.

Until two days ago . . .

Friday afternoon, without so much as an appointment or by your leave, that pushy woman who identified herself as Judine Kelso from Bullion, Inc., International, had been ushered into his office. He scurried around to find a place for her to sit.

Finally seated, Judine asked innocuously, "You're wondering why I came?"

Striving manfully to mask his extreme irritation at this invasion of his domain, he answered sarcastically, "The thought did occur to me. Who are you and why are you here?"

She smiled, not unpleasantly, "All of this material you're digging through originated in my laboratory . . ."

"Oh?" he riposted, "should I stand up and cheer?"

Ignoring his barb, she went on, "And, as you might imagine, BII is extremely desirous of a quick response to my NDA."

Ralston, stared at the woman. "You must be out of your mind. It's been only a couple of months . . ."

"I know, I know," Judine said, "but Oncoplex is a product the world has been waiting for . . ."

He grinned sardonically. "That's what they all say."

"And we thought, that is, BII's chairman of the board and I thought . . . that you might try to move it along a little bit faster than normally . . ."

He stared at her again, his ire rising. "Look, Miss Kelso, all this stuff has to be evaluated and . . ."

While he was talking Judine had been rummaging in the huge bag she carried and pulled out a single sheet of paper and handed it to him. Ralston turned white. "Who gave you this? Where . . . where did you get this?"

Instead of answering, Judine arose and said, "With your permission, Dr. Ralston, I'd like to meet you day after tomorrow and discuss the Oncoplex project in more detail. Where would you like me to meet you?"

Ralston was still staring at the letter. When he heard her voice he looked up. "Where did you come by this?"

"Let's just say that it came to us fortuitously. You may have it. We have the original. And now, for your answer . . ."

He struggled to his feet. "This is . . . it's . . ."

"Let's be careful of our words, Doctor. Why don't we just say that we will meet right here Sunday afternoon. About three?"

Ralston nodded dumbly.

"Three?" she persisted.

He answered hoarsely, "Yes . . . three."

Long after Judine left, Ralston stared at the sheet of paper. Then he angrily wadded it up, took it with him to the rest-room where he entered a stall, burned it and flushed the ashes down the drain.

When would the pain of that terrible mistake ever go away? he asked himself. Ralston knew he had no choice. He knew that he would have to accede to their demands and push the project through. Then what would he do? He could never practice medicine again, his wife had made certain of that. Because, if he ever did, she would expose him.

The loneliness of his joyless existence swept over him, and for the first time since that awful night, he drank himself insensible.

"He's a capable physician," Roger Keller was reporting to a select committee of the BII Board of Directors the following week. "We checked him out thoroughly."

A murmur of approval went around the long table of BII's plush executive board room.

"Then what?" an elegantly-clad woman asked.

"Then what?" Roger asked. "I'm not sure I quite follow you, Edith."

"After the, ah, NDA has been approved . . . then what about, what's his name, Dr. Ralston?"

"Ah, yes. Good question. That could possibly prove a trifle embarrassing later on. We'll make arrangements for him to . . . shall we say, resign his position at the FDA. The man will take a quiet vacation, then with no fanfare we'll see that he is comfortably located in one of our foreign offices . . ."

General nods of approval around the table.

"Another question, Roger," a youngish man asked.

"Yes, Thomas."

"Did Dr. Ralston give any indication when we could expect Oncoplex to be cleared?"

Keller smiled. "Not exactly. However, he assured us it would be very soon."

Late that same evening on Mulholland Drive, Allen Drury's telephone rang. Out on the veranda, enjoying his third Scotch and soda, Allen picked up his portable phone. "Yes . . ."

Characteristically, Collins got right to the point. "What about Jack . . . is he beginning to dabble in laetrile?"

"Not that I know of."

"And that Ben Rush . . . has he been around again?"

"No. Just that once."

"What do you think he's up to?"

Allen cleared his throat nervously. "I don't know. At least not for sure. He said something about Anne's journal . . ."

Collins exploded. "Anne's journal! What do you mean?"

A trickle of sweat ran down Drury's back. "I knew nothing about a journal. Not till Rush mentioned it . . ."

"Did he say what was in it?"

Despite himself, Drury's voice quavered. "Uh, something about her keeping a record of everything having to do with her professional life. And her career. Some personal things . . ."

"What else?"

"He said she started it when she was in Stanford . . ."

"You're a fool, Al! You should have known about that journal. You should have gotten it from Anne before she died."

"What do you mean, Bert? What're you talking about?"

"Do you know what Rush is going to do with that journal? He's a writer. Y' know that? Who knows how he's going to use the stuff."

So, then, Ben now understood, Anne *had* been interested in laetrile. But, just how much had she known? He realized his wife had been a very private person, but was beginning to realize she was far more private that he had been aware.

Dr. Anne's Journal

She had never spoken of having had close friends. Just the opposite. As far as he knew, Carolyn was the closest. And Carolyn admitted that their relationship, though friendly, had never approached what she would call intimate. Ben personally knew that Anne and her father had never shared a meaningful relationship, at least not as far as Anne was concerned.

Aside from her grandparents — both of them now gone — Ben realized that he alone had been his wife's closest confidante. To whom, then, could he turn to learn more about her?

Only her journal . . .

No, there was yet another source. Her books. He knew how his wife had treasured her books, as did he. Perhaps they could open her mind to him. It was worth a try.

Books were evident in nearly every room of their dwellings. But it was in her cabin office where Anne spent most of her time reading, studying and researching. Stocking up the Land Rover with plenty of fresh food from Ralph's Market in Malibu, Ben drove up to the cabin to spend a few days . . .

Monday morning, after breakfast, he stepped into her office. For the first time ever, he gave her library more than a cursory glance. Not knowing exactly what he was looking for, Ben ran his eyes over the three entire walls of shelved books. The majority of them, he noted, were sets of medical books and bound copies of journals, most of them evidently references.

Weeks before, when he had dusted and cleaned, Ben had seen several dozen new books neatly stacked at the end of her desk and near her reading chair. A few of them, he remembered, had come since her death, but most of them had markers in them, and otherwise bore evidence of having been read or at least opened.

Perhaps in these books, Anne's closest and
dearest friends, he would learn what she had been
reading and thinking those last months before she
left him . . .

At random, he picked up a few and read their
titles. His heart gave a lurch. The majority of these
books bore titles relating to the subjects of cancer.
And healing. Some titles and their authors were
familiar to him. Others not.

It looked as though he had hit pay dirt.

One of the first he saw was by an author
whose name he knew: Bernie Siegel, M.D. — *Love,
Medicine and Miracles*. The book bore mute evidence
of having been carefully read. The jacket was worn
and torn in places.

Many passages were underlined, a few of
which he read. One stopped him and he reread it
several times with a growing sense of anguish.

He picked up others, read the titles and
restacked them to be read later — *Recalled By Life,
The Story of My Recovery From Cancer*, by Anthony
J. Sattilaro, M.D. and *Nutrition, The Cancer Answer*,
by Maureen Salaman. *The Cancer Syndrome*, by
Ralph Moss caught his eye. It fell open to a chapter
titled, "The Laetrile Controversy," that was heavily
marked and annotated. He placed that book by itself.

Then, several books in a row joined Moss's
book — *What The Medical Establishment Won't Tell
You That Could Save Your Life*, and *Freedom From
Cancer*, both by medical journalist, Michael L. Culbert
and both with extensive information on laetrile and
related metabolic therapies, much of it highlighted by
Anne.

From the stack beside Anne's desk, Ben chose
a handful of others: *Crackdown on Cancer*, by Ruth
Yale Long, Ph.D.; *Laetrile Case Histories, The
Richardson Cancer Clinic Experience*, by John A.
Richardson, M.D.; and *Murder by Injection, The Story
of the Medical Conspiracy Against America*, by

Dr. Anne's Journal

Eustace Mullins; *Third Opinion, An International Directory to Alternative Therapy Centers for the Treatment and Prevention of Cancer*, by John M. Fink; *Alternative Cancer Therapies, Tijuana Clinics, Where and How To Go*, by Sally Wolper; and *Male Practice*, by Robert S. Mendelsohn, M.D.[28]

Ben surveyed the literal "heaped up evidence" at his feet and knew beyond a wisp of doubt that Anne Rush had been quite well informed concerning laetrile and all other metabolic cancer therapies. Why, he asked himself again, hadn't she availed herself of those alternatives?

He lugged his small stack of books to his reading chair in front of the fireplace. Though the day was not cold, he shivered, which he often did when he was excited or stressed. He quickly laid a fire and touched a match. Warming himself before the open blaze, Ben realized for the first time that there were evil forces beyond his ken that had negatively influenced his wife, ultimately resulting in her death by default . . .

Again he renewed his determination to unearth who or what they were and to deal with them.

CHAPTER TWENTY-TWO

Ben was deeply engrossed in reading Anne's books when he was startled by the telephone. He was even more startled with the first words he heard.

"Hello, Ben," the friendly-sounding voice boomed, ". . . this is Bert Collins. How are you?"

Cautiously, coolly, Ben responded. "Hello, Bert. I'm fine."

"We haven't communicated for a while. Thought I'd just give you a call . . ."

Ben didn't know what to say, so he said nothing. Never in the years that Ben had known the man, had Bert ever initiated *any* communication with him.

"You've written a couple of mighty good books, Ben. I've read them both . . ."

"Thanks . . ." Ben said. What was the man getting at?

"I've just been thinking, Ben . . . Anne was my only child. And I don't have any recent photos of her. Do you have one you could send me?"

Ben furrowed his brow in concentration. A photo? What would the man want with a photo? "Well . . . I guess I could do that."

"And while you're at it . . ."

Ben felt himself tense up in preparation for what was coming next . . .

". . . did Anne keep a diary?"

Dr. Anne's Journal

So, *that* was it, Ben thought. Her journal. "No, not that I've ever seen," he said truthfully.

"Or a journal of some sort?" Collins went on.

Momentarily Ben thought to deny the journal's existence, but thought better of it. "She kept a journal. Mostly a professional, medical journal. Why?"

"Because . . ." Collins began, then hesitated, apparently choosing his words carefully, "because, it would make a wonderful keepsake, a remembrance of my daughter . . ."

The unmitigated gall! Ben thought. The man clearly had desired no contact with his daughter while she was living — and now that she is gone . . .

Bitter words rose in his throat, but he suppressed them. No, he would not give the man the satisfaction of knowing he had angered him. Instead, he chose a temporizing tactic. "I've been reading Anne's journal myself," he said. "It's a very personal journal . . . much of it written during the years that Anne and I knew each other . . . and I intend to keep it myself . . ."

"Don't you think that's being a little selfish? After all, she was my daughter," Collins grated.

Curbing the desire to lash out at the man, Ben said gently, "Your daughter, Mr. Collins, yes. Though I'm not sure that Anne ever felt that you considered her as being worthy of your love. But Anne was *my* wife. And I . . ."

His voice suddenly harsh, Collins said, "Look, Ben, she was my daughter. I raised her, fed and clothed her. Sent her to the best schools, gave her everything . . ."

"Everything except yourself, Mr. Collins . . ."

"Enough of this word play, Rush. Look, that journal of Anne's is important to me. And I intend to have it . . ."

If Collins had more to say, Ben never knew. In the middle of the man's harangue, Ben lowered the phone into its cradle.

After his anger cooled and he ceased trembling, Ben prepared himself a sandwich and resumed his reading.

The "laetrile war," Ben learned, was a war within a war. On December 23, 1971, President Richard Nixon gave to the United States what was to have been one of the greatest Christmas gifts of all time. That was the date when he signed the National Cancer Act into law, thus officially launching what was described as a full-scale assault upon the dread disease.

Congress had designated the Act "a national crusade *to be accomplished* by 1976 in commemoration of the 200th anniversary of our country." To do this, President Nixon called for "the same kind of concentrated effort that split the atom and took man to the moon."[29]

That's been over 14 years, Ben mused, and today more people are dying of cancer than ever before in history. It seems that medicine — at least *orthodox* medicine — in their own words, admits, "... *we are losing the war against cancer.*"[30]

But, he asked himself, has the total war been lost?

Answers to his question, from the alternative therapy camp, was a clear-cut no! To his surprise Ben found himself reading statements such as the one by Dr. Otto Warburg, two-time winner of the Nobel Prize, and others, "There is no disease whose prime cause is better known," and, "Cancer is not the mysterious disease we have been led to believe. You can prevent cancer; it's surprisingly easy. Thousands are doing it."[31]

CHAPTER TWENTY-THREE

"Establishment medicine, call it *orthodox* medicine if you want to, has done a number on us," Ben said.

Bristling slightly, Jack returned, "Do you know what you're talking about?"

"Yes, I do. And I'm learning more every day."

Wednesday morning, after a full day and nearly a full night reading Anne's books, Ben had called Jack. "I think I've got some stuff that'll interest you . . . can we meet?"

"Sure. When? Where?"

"Wherever. Your place? I'm on wheels. You name it and the time and I'll be there."

"Okay. My place. Here's the address. How about seven-thirty this evening?"

"Super. I'll bring some sandwiches . . ."

"Mind if I invite Earl Bailey, my partner?"

"Does he think like you about orthodox medicine?"

"Pretty much."

"Okay," Ben said, "the more the merrier."

Now the three of them were seated in the tiny conference room at Jack's and Earl's clinic in East Los Angeles. Ben passed the sandwiches around and while the others were digging into them, he opened his familiar yellow, lined note pad.

"Just for starters," Ben said, "let me ask you a question." Without waiting for their affirmation, he went on, "How much do either one of you know about the economics of cancer?"

Jack swallowed a bite and said, "Not much . . ."

"And you, Earl," Ben addressed the chiropractor.

"About the same. Very little."

"Okay, let me give you a bit of history . . ."

"I imagine that both of you have heard of the Memorial Sloan Kettering Cancer Institute of New York . . .?"

Both men nodded.

"Okay, and I don't know how much you know about MSKCI, or simply S-K, as it is called, so this might come as a surprise to you, but MSKCI, has been called the 'Temple of the modern method of cancer treatment in the United States.'. . ."[32]

For the next half hour Ben reviewed some of his research with the two doctors. He related the background of the cancer "industry" — and how it centers basically around S-K. In the beginning, the hospital that eventually became S-K, was called Women's Hospital, a 30-bed, all charity hospital. The owner of this hospital, which opened May 1, 1855, on New York's Madison Avenue, was Dr. J. Marion Sims.

Sims, Ben shared with Bailey and Drury, called himself a "women's doctor," who for many years dabbled in operations on slave women in the South he called "experimental surgery." Early in his practice, the man purchased a 17-year-old slave girl named Anarcha for $500, upon whom he performed thirty some operations, without anesthesia.

Jack shuddered. "That's hard to believe . . ."

"I agree," Ben said. "The man's biographer called those operations little short of murderous. He must have been an evil genius. At any rate, he was a genius . . .

"Because," he went on, "when a member of the John Jacob Astor family died of cancer, the family decided to establish a cancer hospital in New York. They approached Sims with an offer of a donation of $150,000 if the Women's Hospital would be turned into a cancer hospital . . ."

An opportunist, Sims had double-crossed the trustees of Women's Hospital, and negotiated privately with the Astors himself. They backed him in creating a new hospital he named the New York Cancer Hospital. Sims, however, died shortly before the hospital opened in 1884.

"A few years later, somewhere in the 1890s," Ben said, "after receiving donations and gifts from other benefactors, the New York Cancer Hospital was renamed Memorial Hospital.

"All of that information might be a little boring," Ben admitted, "but, it's important. Because, in the mid-twentieth century the names Sloan and Kettering were added. Nevertheless, names aside, for many years this cancer center has been one of the appendages of the Rockefeller financial institutions . . ."[33]

"You mean the Rockefellers are tied in with the Sloan-Kettering Cancer Institute?" Earl asked.

"That's right," Ben said, "and S-K considers itself to be *the* leading cancer research center . . . it's a very powerful institution."[34]

"Come off it," Jack said. "No institution is that powerful!"

"Oh?" Ben questioned, "are you actually naive enough to believe that?"

"I resent that!"

"Alright, Jack, go ahead and resent it," Ben said evenly. "But, let me ask you this: Why do you think your father fired you from his practice?"

Jack jumped up and grabbed his coat. "That's a little too much, Ben. You're out of line . . ." Speaking to Earl, he said, "Go ahead and listen to this if you like. But I've had enough. I'm going home . . ."

Earl Bailey just shrugged as Jack pounded out and slammed the door behind him.

Ben said softly, "Earl, I'm sorry to upset Jack like that, but I think I know what I'm talking about."

"I believe you do, Ben. I really think you do . . ."

Later that evening, Carolyn got a call from Ben. "Is it too late to invite you out to dinner?" he asked.

She laughed. "Yes . . . and no."

"Yes it's too late?" he responded. "Or no, it's not too late?"

"The answer is, yes, it's too late for me to go out to dinner. No, it's not too late for you to come here . . ."

"Shall I bring something?"

"Yes, two things?"

"Such as?" he asked.

"First, your appetite. I'll have a huge salad ready for you when you get here . . ."

"And the second?"

She laughed again. "You've got to tell me how you managed to get Jack so upset . . ."

"It's a deal. I'm as hungry as a horse. And, as for Jack, I've got some very interesting information to share with you — that he didn't stick around to hear."

An hour later, Ben sighed contentedly and folded his napkin. "Carolyn, that's a much better meal than I make. Thanks."

"You're welcome. First, I'll clear the table, then I'll be ready for the interesting information you promised . . ."

Carolyn took Ben's hand and led him to the balcony that overlooked the marina. Companionably they followed the port and starboard running lights of a few late-returning boats as they belatedly made their way into the harbor. Beyond the marina, an almost steady stream of air traffic was landing and taking off from Los Angeles International Airport.

Venus was brightly watching overhead . . .

"Sunset and evening star . . ." Carolyn whispered.

Ben tensed briefly, remembering Anne, then relaxed and finished the stanza, ". . . and let there be no moaning at the bar when I put out to sea . . ."

She smiled up into his face, and he momentarily resisted the urge to hold her. Then she was in his arms. Warm. Gentle. Alive. He kissed her softly. She lingered for a moment, then moved away. "That was nice, Ben . . . very nice."

She shivered. "It's cool. Let's go inside . . . I'll put on a sweater and be ready for the promised information . . ."

Ben was surprised to find himself trembling, and was glad for the moment she was gone to regain control. Then she was back, vivacious, smiling . . .

"Okay, Ben . . . you're on . . ."

He nodded. "Well, for beginners, I've just learned something that was news to me. You may already have known it. Or at least suspected it. The so-called fight against cancer is not a fight at all . . .

"Cancer research, for the most part, is not an open market as we might suppose. Or would like to believe. Because, much of it is bogus. And there is little doubt but that it is totally controlled by the cancer establishment . . ."[35]

Carolyn raised her eyebrows. "Cancer establishment? That sounds like a well-organized cartel . . . a conspiracy . . ."

"I agree. And that's the very question Senator Edward Kennedy put to Dr. John Richardson . . .?"

"Oh? What was the answer?"

"Dr. Richardson answered, 'I definitely feel that there is. Yes.'[36] Senator Kennedy responded by asking, 'Who is involved in this conspiracy?'"

The very possibility of such a conspiracy chilled Carolyn and she shivered, pulling her sweater more tightly around her shoulders. She could not resist another question. "How did Dr. Richardson respond?"

Ben answered slowly. "Richardson named various organizations interested in the cancer field: the American Cancer Society, the Food and Drug Administration, the American Medical Association, and the Sloan Kettering Institute . . ."[37]

"Does anyone else support Dr. Richardson's charges?"

"Yes, among them, G. Edward Griffin, who is well known for his numerous documentary books and films. Among other statements on the subject, Griffin speaks of a 'malicious conspiracy hiding behind the smiling mask of humanitarianism . . .'"[38]

Giving Carolyn a moment to digest this information, Ben went on, "Besides, it's become increasingly clear to me — and should be to anyone interested in digging for the facts — that the cancer industry is actually an industry like any other. And the bottom line is, in one word: profits . . ."

Carolyn gasped. "You can't mean that."

"Sorry, Carolyn, but I do mean it. Until 1945, Memorial Hospital — now the Memorial Sloan-Kettering Cancer Center — was under the control of the Rockefellers, and to a lesser degree, the Douglasses. Since that time MSKCC has become the world's largest private cancer center and is now ruled by what looks like a consortium of Wall Street's top banks and corporations . . ."[39]

Chapter Twenty-Three

"Okay, Ben, take the wheel," Ross said. "I'm going to shake out the jib. Hold her steady on 270 degrees till we get out a few miles . . ."

The two of them were just clearing the breakwater of the Marina Del Rey marina and heading out to the open sea. The *Blue Pencil* was a sprightly sloop and behaved like a colt let out to pasture. The knife-sharp bow split the blue water cleanly, leaving a crisp, foaming bow wave.

I'm glad I came along, Ben thought.

After leaving Carolyn's condo, Ben decided to stay in Santa Monica that night instead of returning to Malibu. He realized he was suffering from "information shock," and wanted to talk it over with Ross Hannibal. He knew Ross was an early riser, so he called him at home instead of the office.

"I was going to take the day off and go sailing," Ross told him. "You just caught me going out the door . . ."

"Oh . . . might I see you at your office tomorrow?"

"Why not at my office at the marina?"

"Marina?"

"Yeah, sure. The marina. Meet me on board the *Blue Pencil*. That's what I call my marina office."

"Well . . . I don't want to spoil your day . . ."

"Spoil it, nothing. Come and go along with me. I've got enough food packed for the two of us . . ."

Now, on board the *Blue Pencil*, his jib tended to, Ross made his way carefully back to the cockpit where he broke out the cucumber and tomato sandwiches and apple cider he had brought along.

The sloop heeled over in the freshening breeze and Ben held the wheel with both hands, keeping an eye on the foot of the sail to keep it from luffing. "Good going, Ben," Ross said. "I can see you've done this before . . ."

"Not for several years . . . but I love it."

"We'll have to do this more often . . ."

Finally clear of the early morning marina channel traffic, Ross settled himself comfortably. "Okay, Ben, what is it you wanted to talk about — that just wouldn't wait?"

"There's so much to tell . . . but, before I get into that, I've got a question . . ."

"Which is?" Ross asked quietly, bracing himself against the rolling swell of the open sea.

"Just how much do you want me to tell?"

"You'll have to be more specific."

Ben drew in a deep breath of the freshening breeze and eased up on the wheel. "The cancer story . . . the frauds, the ripoff, the pharmaceutical cartel . . . the medical industrial complex? How much do we dare to publish?"

Ross chuckled. "How much've you got?"

"A lot . . ."

"All of it having to do with freedom of choice in medicine?"

"All of it. Either directly or indirectly . . ."

Ross wiped spray from his face and took a sip of cider. He chose his words carefully. "Let me remind you again of Cutting Edge's editorial philosophy. Our company was formed for the specific purpose of exposing medical and pharmaceutical malpractice, conspiracy and fraud wherever it exists. That's our reason for being. Does that answer your question?"

Ben nodded. "I just wanted to hear it from you again."

"Okay, Ben, then here it is for the record, let's do it up right. Give us all of it. As much as you can document and still hold the interest of the public. So they can check it out."

Ben thought about that. He shifted the wheel a couple of notches to hold the *Blue Pencil* on course. He squinted in the bright sun as he turned to Ross.

"Okay, Ross. Okay . . . I'll do my best to give them the facts *and* make it palatable."

The fire engines roared past, siren blaring and bells jangling. Ben groaned and stuffed the pillow around his head to cut out the noise. The jangling bells continued. Suddenly he realized he'd been asleep. His telephone was ringing . . .

He fumbled and picked it up. "Yes . . ." he managed.

"Oh, Mr. Rush . . . it's late. I apologize . . ."

"Uh, that's all right . . ." he yawned. "I just got to sleep. Been a long day . . ."

"Please forgive me, but aren't you the man Dr. Richardson's secretary told me about? Who's writing a book on cancer . . .?"

Suddenly fully awake, Ben sat up. "Yes, Miss . . ."

"It's Mrs. . . . Mrs. Klinger. From Montana . . . from Kalispel, Montana . . ."

"Oh, oh, yes. Well, Mrs. Klinger, you're right. I am writing a book. But not just about cancer. It's about cancer therapies . . . alternative therapies . . ."

"Oh, that's good. Because, that's what I wanted to talk about. You see, I had cancer. Terminal cancer. Fourteen years ago. My doctor in Montana gave me up and told me he couldn't do anything more for me . . ."

"Fourteen years ago? What happened?"

"Well, I heard about Dr. Richardson in California. He had an office in Albany, California at the time . . ."

Ben grabbed his yellow writing pad. "Richardson? Dr. John Richardson?"

"Yes . . . he's a wonderful man. Before I went to him they had just about killed me . . . mastectomy. Metastasized. They removed eleven lymph nodes . . . gave me 4,500 rads of cobalt therapy, and . . ."

Ben was writing furiously. "Forty-five hundred? Did you say 4,500 rads of cobalt?"

"Yes, sir. They about killed me. Then I was told that was all they could give me. They gave me hormones . . . didn't do any good. The cancer came back again . . ."

Ben could hear the woman crying. "It was awful . . . I had a husband and two small children . . . and I was dying . . ."

"What happened?" Ben asked softly. "Something good must have happened. Tell me about it."

"Well, like I said, I went to the Richardson Cancer Clinic, the one they closed up. That was a terrible shame. I believe lots of people died when they closed him down. Anyway, Dr. Richardson gave me what he called metabolic therapy . . ."

"Explain that for me, please . . ."

"Well, vitamins, minerals and enzymes. Good nutrition — lots of fresh fruit and vegetables. And, of course, regular amounts of laetrile. I still take laetrile to this day . . ."

"Mrs. Klinger," Ben said, "please listen very carefully. Do you have all of your hospital and doctor records . . .?"

"Oh, yes. All of them. You can have them if you want them. I just want to let people know that no matter how bad you might get . . . if you've got faith . . ."

"And a good doctor," Ben interjected.

"Yes, sir, I was just going to say that. If you've got faith and a good doctor who doesn't overdose you with drugs and with that terrible, that awful, awful chemotherapy . . . well, then, there's hope . . ."

"Mrs. Klinger, I can't tell you how grateful I am for your call . . ."

"I'm glad I caught you, Mr. Rush. I'll send all my X-rays and records to you tomorrow. I'm just glad that somebody is writing a book like you are. I hope I can see a copy when it comes out . . ."[40]

"You will, Mrs. Klinger. Believe me, you will . . ."

Ben tried to go back to sleep, but couldn't. His mind was so filled to capacity with all he'd been learning the past few days that even when he closed his eyes an endless stream of words kept flowing across the screen of his mind.

After turning and twisting for another hour, he got up, brewed himself a cup of herbal tea and went to his computer. By the time the sun rose over Santa Monica bay, Ben had written the synopsis he had promised Ross Hannibal.

Jack Drury was still angry when he got to the clinic the next morning. There was a note on his door for him to telephone his father. Apprehensive, he slowly punched Allen Drury's office number. Carolyn answered, her usual cheerful self.

But, for once, he didn't feel like talking to her. Yes, she told him, his father was in. Yes, he was expecting Jack to call and she would buzz him.

"Hello, Dad . . . you wanted me to call."

"Yes, Jack. A lot has happened since I talked to you last."

"Oh, what's that?"

Allen used his best patient, bedside manner tone. "Remember, what I asked you then? To shy away from anything — anything *or* anybody — that had to do with that so-called alternative stuff?"

"Yes, Dad . . . I remember . . ." He felt his muscles tense. "Why . . . what's up?"

"Okay, Jack, we differed on alternative medicine . . . and chiropractors . . . and drugs. That's all water under the bridge. Now things are getting serious. It's out of my hands. I've been told to tell you . . ." he struggled to keep control.

Dr. Anne's Journal

"Jack, believe me, you've got to stay away from alternative therapies . . . and everything and anybody that has to do with them . . ."

"Wait a minute, Dad. What's this all about?"

"That's all I can tell you, Son . . ."

"Wait a minute, Dad. Don't hang up?"

The senior Drury answered in a choking voice. "What is it, Jack?"

"Please tell me what this is all about? Why are you telling me this . . . but not the rest of it?"

"Jack, please, don't ask me anything more. Just do what I say. I want to help you . . . but . . . but, there's only so much I can do. All I can tell you is this . . . if you don't watch your step, you could lose your license . . . goodbye."

A very sober Jack Drury hung up his telephone.

CHAPTER TWENTY-FOUR

As she opened and read the letter, Judine Kelso's hands began trembling. This was her third such letter in less than a month. One of the FDA requirements before licensing new drugs was the testing of the drugs on both animals and humans. Kelso had already successfully tested Oncoplex on animals and the majority of reports were positive in every respect. According to her lab records, "In 98% of the animals tested, Oncoplex inhibited and caused rejection of induced or transplanted tumors."

"Furthermore," she noted, "during the testing period, not a single female conceived. In the same manner in which Oncoplex prevented the cancer cells from finding refuge in the host, and were thus rejected and expelled from the body, fertilized ovum in the tested animals were prevented from implanting in the uterus and were consequently rejected."

By now, the project was in Phase III of the testing program. In this phase Oncoplex was administered to cancer patients under fully monitored conditions, as similar as possible to the same conditions projected in later use. Up till now, reports had been mostly positive and uniformly good.

Except for these three letters.

The letters had come from three widely-separated hospitals chosen for testing. Each letter had been careful to state that Oncoplex had been used only under strictly controlled conditions, in each case with the patients' signed permission, which were usually not difficult to obtain.

All three of the letters recounted essentially the same story. On the majority of cancer patients within the control group, on which Oncoplex was used, the drug had acted true to form and massive numbers of cancer cells were excreted; the results Judine's animal studies had projected. Even the expected side effects — nausea and vomiting, elevated blood pressure, dizziness and diarrhea — were minimal. So far so good.

However, Judine read with growing apprehension, all three of the hospitals reported unexpected incidents of uncontrollable diarrhea, fever and runaway high blood pressure. The symptoms came on suddenly and did not respond to palliative measures. Patients quickly slipped into a coma and expired within a few hours without regaining consciousness.

Already, during the year of human testing, several thousand patients had received Oncoplex with only positive results. But now, all at once, *three patients had died.*

Three, but *only* three, out of thousands. Judine was a scientist and knew that it was possible for these fatalities to be a mere fluke, a rare and unusual occurrence, having absolutely no connection with Oncoplex. Possible . . .

There was little doubt as to the overall efficacy of this new drug, and that it would prove to be an extremely beneficial drug, one that would undoubtedly save many lives. She knew it was her duty to report these fatalities to the FDA. But to do so would result in setting back the launching of Oncoplex for at least another full year.

Already BII had spent millions on the publicity plans in anticipation of the approval of "the cancer-fighting drug of the century." Judine was in a dilemma. Actually a double dilemma. Not only did

BII have a vested interest in Oncoplex, but she did. It was her baby. She had conceived it and nurtured it throughout its very long gestation period. Now it was ready for birth. And could she abort her own child?

What should she do? Tell Keller? File the letters and tell nobody? After several sleepless nights, she decided to suppress the information and do nothing . . .

Within a short period of time, with the cooperation of Dr. Ralston, Oncoplex's application was approved.

The Federal Drug Administration's decision regarding another substance that they chose to take under their jurisdiction was handled in an entirely different manner. That substance, Ben was learning, was laetrile.

To his utter amazement Ben learned that laetrile is in legal limbo in the United States. Labeling it as an "unlicensed new drug," the FDA has outlawed the substance, making it unlawful to import or to ship across state lines. Beyond that, laetrile's use is opposed by most of the medical establishment.

Based on the Establishment's official position that laetrile is a "worthless, harmless substance," their rationale for taking such drastic action against its use is unclear.

So, for Anne, a physician, it could have been argued that she possessed valid *professional* reasons for refusing treatment with laetrile. If that, indeed, was her reason, she was not in the minority. Thousands of doctors faced with the controversies surrounding laetrile — or amygdalin, or Vitamin B-17 — and the fear tactics utilized by its opponents, refused to have anything to do with it.

But Anne? Had she shied away from laetrile because of controversy? Or were there other reasons?

Dr. Anne's Journal

"This whole field of medicine is new to me," Ben was saying, "but when my wife died of lymphoma, I was left with a long list of unanswered questions . . ."

"I think we've all got a lot of those."

The two of them were seated in Michael Culbert's ample office in Chula Vista, about halfway between San Diego and the Mexican border. Like a typical editor's office, it was crammed with file cabinets and books.

As Ben had become more knowledgeable in the field, names that had previously meant nothing to him when he first read them in Anne's journal now took on flesh and blood, and assumed lives of their own. Names such as Dr. John A. Richardson . . . By her journal entries, Ben now realized that Anne was at least somewhat acquainted with Richardson and had corresponded with him on more than one occasion.

She knew that Richardson had fought a bitter court battle with the powers that be over his freedom to treat his patients as he saw fit. In one of her journal entries Anne quoted a few lines from the State Code under which all California physicians are licensed, and which Richardson had used in his own defense . . .

> *Nothing in this chapter shall be construed so as to discriminate against any particular school of medicine or surgery, school of podiatry, or any other treatment. . . .*[41]

Obviously, Richardson believed he was within his rights to use any method of treatment, regardless of the school of medical thought behind it. He had merely acted in accordance with his conscience and professional expertise when he ministered to his patients. Even so, Richardson's stand eventually resulted in the loss of his medical license.

Had Anne feared the same result?

Another name that cropped up frequently in Anne's journal was Michael L. Culbert, D.Sc. She possessed at least two of his books and had apparently been in contact with him.

Culbert, Ben learned, was the editor of *The Choice*, "The International Newsmagazine of Metabolic Therapy and Freedom of Choice in Medicine," as well as Chairman of the Board and Director of Public Relations for American Biologics-Mexico S.A. Medical Center.[42] American Biologics, or AB, is a leader in individualized, integrated metabolic programs and eclectic medicine and occupies a new, modern, fully-equipped in- and out-patient facility, a mere 30-minute drive south of San Diego.

After spending a couple of hours reading Culbert's books and magazine, it was obvious that the man was and had been deeply involved in the freedom of choice battle from the outset. Perhaps he could supply some answers to Ben's growing list of questions.

Culbert's office number was listed on the masthead of *The Choice*. On impulse, Ben picked up his telephone and dialed it.

After chatting a couple of minutes, Ben asked if they could meet. Culbert was agreeable. Could Ben come to Chula Vista? Yes, he could come the next day . . .

Ben caught an early flight to San Diego and rented a car. By 10:00 a.m., he drove up to the American Biologics' inauspicious office. Michael Culbert, wearing his habitual safari suit, was expecting him.

"Today is my day to go to our clinic in Tijuana," Mike was saying. "I thought you might like to go along, so I planned the day accordingly . . ."

Dr. Anne's Journal

"My time is my own," Ben said. "And I'd very much like to go with you."

Culbert, Ben already knew, had been a newsman for nearly thirty years, with an impressive list of credits. In addition to having served as editor of a Venezuelan newspaper, the *Berkeley Daily Gazette* and the *Richmond Independent* newspapers, he had been a magazine correspondent, a stringer for *Time*, *Life* and NBC and had produced his own radio commentary show.

"How did you make the transition from newspaperman to your present position?" Ben asked, when they got on the freeway.

"Well, I guess it just happened . . ." he chuckled.

It seemed that Culbert, the then editor of the *Berkeley Daily Gazette* during the early 70s had had no choice but to cover the happenings of "Laetrile movement" that was erupting in his territory.

"As a journalist," he said, "I was skeptical of Laetrile. But, as I dug into the situation, I was frustrated because I couldn't get any straight answers to two important questions — questions I still don't have answers for . . ."

"What are they?" Ben asked.

"The first one is this: What right does government have to interfere with the doctor-patient relationship and deny the doctor and the patient access to Laetrile, or any other modality or substance they desire for the healing process? Denial of that opportunity would seem to be criminal . . . especially when that patient has been described as terminal, and all orthodox remedies have failed."

Ben shook his head. "It's unfair, I agree . . ."

"And the second one is just as pertinent: Why should honest Americans be treated like criminals? Why should they be forced to go underground . . . or flee the country to secure a treatment such as laetrile? At the worst it's described by some as being 'worthless' — but it's almost always admitted to be harmless."

"You mean, by trying to get the answers to those questions you got involved?"

Mike grinned. "That's about it . . . you see, I knew Dr. Richardson. At least I knew who he was. He was an honorable, well thought of doctor in the community. He was doing a lot of good. And when the district attorney told me he was going to bust him, I said, 'Look out. That case will blow up in your hands.'"

Mike grinned, remembering. "And he did. And it did."

Being a weekday, the U.S./Mexico Border crossing was not crowded with tourists, and within minutes they were in Mexico.

"Oh, before I forget to ask," Ben began, "you undoubtedly know something about Linus Pauling . . .?"

Linus Pauling, Ben knew, now nearing the ripe young age of 90, is one of the world's greatest living scientists, and one of a small handful of persons to have received not one, but two Nobel prizes. Despite the numerous accolades laid at this genial giant's feet, including the fact that he is doubtless the world's acknowledged expert on Vitamin C, Pauling is unable to elicit a grant for cancer research from the Cancer Establishment.

The reason: Pauling believes and promulgates the thesis that cancer is connected with nutrition. He makes no bones about his position, and it has cost him dearly, literally drying up the funds the Pauling Institute desperately needs.

Based on two decades of research, Pauling publicly stated his opinion in an ad in the *Wall Street Journal*, "Our research shows that the incidence and severity of cancer depends upon diet. We urgently want to refine that research, so that it may help to decrease suffering from human cancer. . . ."[43]

Anne had copied Pauling's statement in her journal. When he came across it, Ben was reminded of the dinner table discussion she and he had had about Linus Pauling.

"His ideas on nutrition and Vitamin C run counter to those currently held by practically every doctor I know . . ."

"Meaning what?" Ben asked. "That they're right and he's wrong? Or vice versa?"

"I don't know, Ben. I wish I did know. But, it's difficult to argue with his logic. After all, he is a chemist . . . and he has won a Nobel Prize in chemistry. He also discovered the cause of sickle-cell anemia . . ."

"It seems that I remember he won another Nobel Prize for peace in, what was it, 1962?"

"I believe so. But, the point is . . . Pauling is *not* a medical doctor, and what he is saying really infringes on medical territory . . ."

"So you're not sure if you can accept his conclusions?"

Anne nodded. "You realize, Ben, everyone — even doctors — see only what they are trained to see. For example, if you're unaware of nutritional diseases, you'd never be able to see them, even when they stare you full in the face. Understand?"

"Yes. It makes sense . . ."

She shrugged. "So, I think that's about the size of it."

Ben had to remember that Anne was a physician, and as a member of that elite profession, had great difficulty in accepting the opinions of the "outsiders," especially as they applied to her chosen field of endeavor. It was an occupational hazard not uncommon among the ranks of any profession.

But Linus Pauling?

He was truly an eclectic scientist and certainly could not be charged with having his head in the sand. "I believe," Dr. Linus Pauling said, "that the main objective of cancer treatment should be to give the patient a long, useful, comfortable, contented, productive, and satisfying life."

Following that statement, Dr. Pauling spoke of and listed a number of different kinds of treatment available to achieve the above desirable outcomes, including hormone therapy, immunotherapy, general supportive measures, supplemental ascorbate (Vitamin C) and what he classed generally as "other nutritional or unconventional treatments, *used either alone or in various combinations.*"[44]

Pauling, Ben learned, had a great deal to say about the immune system. As it does with all other forces bent on destroying the body, Pauling pointed out that the immune system "acts as a police force, continually patrolling the tissues, detecting any miscreants and then destroying them, and in this way keeping the body free from cancer. . . .

"Thus," Pauling declared, "enhancing the immune system could play an important part in general cancer treatment, and any measure that depresses the immune system (and unfortunately cancer chemotherapy does just that) decreases the effectiveness of treatment."[45]

But how, Ben asked himself, does one go about enhancing the immune system?

Again, Pauling offered a possible solution.

As a result of his extensive research, Pauling observed that "cancer patients generally exhibit a decreased effectiveness of their natural immune protective mechanisms and almost invariably have a low ascorbate (Vitamin C) content in their lymphocytes (cancer-fighting white blood cells)."

In relation to that fact, Pauling made a powerful statement that caused Ben to pause and consider:

Dr. Anne's Journal

"The simplest and safest way to enhance immunocompetence in these patients . . ." Pauling said, "is to increase their intake of Vitamin C. Only when the increased demand for and utilization of Vitamin C in cancer are fully satisfied can these immune mechanisms provide the maximum protection against the wayward cancer cell."[46]

All of this information was behind the question Ben had just put to Mike Culbert . . .

Culbert didn't hesitate. "Do I know about Linus Pauling? Of course. He's a living legend. Why?"

"Does he have anything to say on the subject of laetrile?"

"Yes. In fact, he's quite vocal on the subject. He makes the statement — as do most therapists who use or advocate the use of laetrile — that what is called 'laetrile treatment of cancer' is of benefit to most cancer patients . . ."

"That's very interesting," Ben said.

"However," Mike when on, "there's more to his statement than meets the eye."

"What's that?"

"Linus Pauling observes that what is commonly called the 'laetrile treatment of cancer' is usually much more than simply giving a patient laetrile . . . and he is right."

As he skillfully wended his way through the Tijuana traffic, Mike spelled out for Ben the basics of laetrile's use in the treating of cancer.

"As you might know," he said, "most physicians who use laetrile either inject it or give it orally. However, and this is extremely important, these cancer patients are usually put on a vegetarian diet, and — along with the laetrile — are given digestive enzymes, minerals, and large amounts or megadoses of vitamins, including vitamins A and C. Vitamin C is usually prescribed in the amount of 10 grams per day."[47]

"That's a lot of Vitamin C," Ben commented.

"Perhaps," Mike agreed, "but Pauling's research has led him to believe that essentially all human beings are suffering from hypoascorbemia, or a deficiency of Vitamin C in the blood. And that the disease can be controlled only by ingesting large amounts of Vitamin C every day . . ."[48]

Ben was so interested in Mike's impartation of his vast knowledge on the subject, that he was surprised when the car stopped and Mike announced, "Here we are." Ben saw that they had pulled up in front of a neat, two-story building bearing the sign: American Biologics-Mexico S.A. Medical Center.

On his return flight to Los Angeles that evening, Ben had much to ponder. He remembered the American Biologics-Mexico S.A. Clinic as being one of the cleanest, most upbeat and positive health institution he had ever seen. Tijuana and its environs boasts a score or more clinics that treat cancer and other degenerative diseases. Among them, names such as the Manner Clinic, Hospital Ernesto Contreras and Hospital Santa Monica, came immediately to mind.[49]

Almost without exception, Ben now realized, these clinics utilize a wide variety of modalities, often including the use of laetrile. After being diagnosed and treated — depending upon the severity of his case — the patient would be trained and provided with the materials to care for himself, then sent home.

"If a patient is being treated with laetrile," Mike told Ben, "he will receive a prescription for laetrile, and allowed to purchase a few month's supply before he leaves the country . . ."

"But, he can't obtain laetrile in the United States?"

"Yes, and no," Mike said. "It is not illegal to manufacture laetrile in the United States, and I know of at least one state that does so. The problem comes in distribution. The FDA has made it illegal to ship laetrile across state lines."

"Do you mean the cancer patient in need of laetrile must personally go back to Mexico to obtain it?"

"That's right. Even though, as of this moment, the *use* of laetrile is legal in 21 states, it cannot be stocked or sold in those states, *even by physicians*, nor can an American doctor prescribe laetrile for a cancer patient."[50]

"Then, how do you define *legal* in those states?"

"It means that those 21 states have passed laws indicating that they will not prosecute doctors for administering laetrile within those states."

Ben shook his head. "But I don't understand. If the use of laetrile is legal in those states, but the doctor can neither prescribe nor obtain it, of what good is that?"

Mike laughed. "That's the problem. A cancer patient must go to Mexico, obtain a prescription, purchase his laetrile in Mexico — for his own use only — and transport it back to one of those 21 states. There, hopefully, a doctor will inject it for him."

"And if the doctors refuse?"

Mike shrugged. "That's the hard part. That's the question that has no answer . . ."

Retrieving his Land Rover from Lot C, Ben drove to his condo in Santa Monica where a message from Jack Drury awaited him on his answering device. "Please call me, Ben. I owe you an apology and I'd like to make it in person . . ."

Before unpacking, Ben dialed Jack's home number. Jack picked it up on the second ring. "Oh, hi, Ben," he said, coming straight to the point, "can we get together? I think we've got a lot to talk about?"

"Well, I'm heading out to my cabin in Malibu first thing in the morning . . ."

"How about breakfast before you leave?"

Ben thought a moment and made a quick decision. "Tell you what, Jack. If you don't mind driving to Malibu — back in the boonies — I'll prepare us a lunch and we'll have all afternoon. What about it?"

"It's a deal . . . tell me how to get there."

"I don't know all that's happening these days," Jack was saying, "but something mighty weird is going on?"

Jack was watching Ben prepare what they agreed was their favorite meal — grilled fish and salad — in the Malibu cabin kitchen. He had kicked off his shoes, leaned back in his chair, and was enjoying a Perrier, the strongest drink Ben offered.

"Why, what's happening?" Ben asked as he sliced tomatoes and cucumbers. He looked up, "Do you like garlic?"

"Love it. Lots of it." Jack set down his glass. "Well, after I stomped out of the office the other day like a 10-year-old kid . . ."

Ben grinned. "You looked like you could have slugged me."

"Felt like it, too. Anyway, Dad had left a call for me. I called him back. Pretty depressing . . ."

"Oh?" Ben looked up. "How so?"

"Well, he'd been after me to keep away from the alternative therapies . . . for some reason. I didn't know why. He'd even warned me before . . ."

"Warned you? On what grounds?"

"I don't know. He never said. But this time it wasn't like the other times. This time he sounded upset. Scared, really. He told me to back off . . . and when I asked him why, he didn't answer for a minute. Then he said something that really shook me. I mean, *really* shook me . . ."

"In what way?"

"He intimated that if I didn't, that 'they' — and he didn't say who 'they' were — might use their influence to have my medical license revoked . . ."

Ted Shaffer knew he was in trouble the morning he awakened with a full bladder, but was unable to urinate. An aeronautical engineer, Ted was generally cool-headed and rarely inclined to panic. The problem had not developed overnight, and Ted's wife had repeatedly urged him to seek medical help. With each flare up, Ted renewed his promise to himself and to her that he would do so. But, with each respite, he soon forgot his good intentions and did nothing . . .

Finally, he *had* gone to a doctor, with terrifying results.

There was something different about this "attack" — he insisted on calling these episodes attacks. More intense, maybe. He couldn't tell for sure. But it *was not* like the others. Despite the somewhat urgent discomfort, he forced himself to calmly put himself through the paces that had proven effective in prior situations . . .

Ted knew he was not alone in this situation. Some of his friends spoke of their difficulties. Some with grim humor. He had laughed with them. "Just age . . . the prostate always goes with age. You get used to it . . ."

Some had joked about prostatic cancer. Not Ted. At least not after his visit to the specialist.

He convinced himself he'd just have to "grin and bear it." That there was nothing else he could do about it. And he had gotten used to it for a time. What was different this time? Trembling, he reached for the pills the man had given him. Sometimes they had helped. But not this time . . .

The difference was: Now he *knew* it was cancer. Prostatic cancer. Just thinking the word filled him with panic.

"No!" he spoke aloud to his image in the mirror, chagrined at the tense, 53-year-old man who stared back at him. "I will not . . . I *will not* allow myself to have cancer. Never. Never!"

As some of his friends had advised, with a supreme act of will, Ted relaxed the muscles of his back and abdomen. No result. He turned on both lavatory faucets full force and waited. No result. Finally, he tried the step that had always worked: he stood in the lukewarm shower and allowed the water to slide across his thighs . . .

The pressure and pain persisted without let up . . .

Thirty minutes had gone by. It was time for him to shave and dress to catch his ride.

"Ted, dear," his wife called from the bottom of the stairs, "Your breakfast is ready. And your ride will soon be here . . ."

"Thanks, Toni . . . be right down."

Even the effort of raising his voice increased the level of pain. He *had to do something*. But what?

The pressure increased. He must have relief. By now sweat was sliding down his back, wrinkling his freshly starched and ironed shirt. His pulse rate accelerated, pounding in his ears. "Oh, God, I can't ride in the car like this . . ."

Sudden decision: "Toni, please come here . . . hurry!"

Her eyes widened. "The same problem?"

He nodded.

"Lie down," she commanded. "Here, on the floor. I'll put a pillow under your hips . . . to help ease the pressure . . ."

He responded quickly, each move generating new shards of pain, that threatened to steal consciousness. He groaned . . .

Dr. Anne's Journal

In the distance, the sound wavering in and out, he heard Toni on the phone. "Dr. Bailey . . . yes. Toni. Toni Shaffer. Please, can you come . . . it's Ted. I believe he's having trouble with his prostate . . .

"Yes, Dr. Bailey, I know you're a chiropractor. But, don't you have a medical doctor on staff with you now? You do? And you'll ask him to come? That's wonderful! Oh, thank you, Dr. Bailey . . . Thank God!"

Jack raised his eyebrows. "Prostate? How did she know that's what it is?"

Earl Bailey shrugged. "I can't tell you. I've treated Ted for back problems for years. He's an engineer. He eats too much. Doesn't exercise. But prostate? He never mentioned it. I don't know. Anyway, I could hear him groaning . . . I told her you'd come . . ."

"Okay, Earl . . . haven't made house calls in a while. But, here goes. I'm on my way . . ."

CHAPTER TWENTY-FIVE

Until his father fired him, Jack Drury's life had been more secure than about anyone he knew. Though he had loved his mother, even his parents' divorce when he was 15 had not terribly shaken him for long. He had become more deeply involved with sports, especially boxing, which had rewarded him with a Golden Gloves trophy and a broken nose that had refused to heal properly.

A hitch in the Navy had completed his medical schooling, and by the time he was 32, Jack was happily practicing medicine with his father in Beverly Hills. Early in his chosen profession Jack realized he felt more drawn to a holistic "wellness" concept of patient care than the more predominant, sickness-oriented, drug-surgery-related modalities currently in vogue.

Naively, Jack supposed that the senior Drury would accept his medical philosophy as being complementary to his own, and that the practice would benefit. He was soon to discover his error and after only two years practicing, together father and son had a parting of ways.

Practicing now with Dr. Earl Bailey, it was evident that the two were successfully melding medical and chiropractic healing modalities into a viable health-providing organization that was being received enthusiastically by their patients.

Dr. Anne's Journal

Ted was rolling on the floor in agony when Jack arrived and quickly checked his vital signs. "I think we should get your husband to the hospital . . ." Jack told Mrs. Shaffer.

"No!" Ted ejaculated. "No hospital . . . just do something to relieve my bladder pressure. And the pain. It's killing me. Please."

"I can catheterize you, Mr. Shaffer. I believe that'll give you temporary relief . . . but if I'm going to really help you I've got to know what's causing the problem."

As he spoke, Jack was opening his bag. Moments later, with the catheter inserted, the pressure was relieved and Ted was up and moving around with little difficulty or pain.

He smiled for the first time that morning. "Dr. Drury, I thank you. I don't believe I could have endured a ride to the hospital . . . would have killed me . . ."

Jack was quietly repacking his bag.

Shaffer said, "Doctor, can you give me something to prevent it from happening again?"

Jack shook his head. "Sit down, Mr. Shaffer. We've got to talk about this . . ." He smiled at Mrs. Shaffer. "You, too, please. This concerns you both."

When they were seated, Ted grinned. "You sound very *serious*, Doctor. I'm feeling fine now. All I need is . . ."

"Wait," Jack said. "Let me give you the facts before you make a decision. First, I've got to know, is this the first time you've had this problem? Or has it happened before ?"

Before Ted could answer, Toni spoke up. "Doctor, Ted's had difficulty like this for quite a while. Not this bad before. And I've begged him to see a doctor . . ."

"Now, Toni, it hasn't been *that* bad . . ."

She went on determinedly. "Yes it has. Not like this, I know. But, you've got to admit you've been having trouble right along. Haven't you?"

He nodded. "Yes . . . you're right." Toni turned to Jack. "What do you think's the problem?"

"I can't tell without a thorough examination . . ."

"But, what *could* it be? Cancer? Prostate cancer?"

Toni gasped.

Jack said evenly. "Mr. Shaffer. I can't rule that out until I examine you. Which is something I will have to do in my office. It might merely be a bladder obstruction of some kind. It might be inflammation of the prostate gland. It could be a number of things. Yes, and to answer your question, it just *could* be cancer of the prostate. But, until I examine you . . ."

Ted digested that for a moment. Then he abruptly arose and stuck out his hand. "Well, Doctor, I thank you for coming. I'll pay you now, or you can bill me . . ." He grinned engagingly. "But I wish you'd write me a prescription or something."

Jack shook his head. "Sorry, not until I know for sure what it's all about."

Toni said, "But, Ted, I don't think you should be going to work today. And I really wish you'd make an appointment."

He grinned. "I tell you, Toni, I'm fine. If it happens again I'll do something. But, right now . . ." he checked his watch. "Anyway, right now I've got to run. Important meeting. Thanks again, Doctor."

Carolyn idly traced geometric designs on her napkin. How does one begin to blow the whistle on one's boss? she asked herself. Across the table from her, Ben waited patiently. Carolyn had called him and asked him to meet at her home for dinner.

"Sure thing," he said, "anytime a good cook asks me to dinner, it's a date . . ."

Dr. Anne's Journal

"It's not really a date," Carolyn told him when they were seated. She indicated the stack of books on the floor.

Ben raised his eyebrows. "It sounds serious. Is it?"

"Yes, very serious . . ."

She began serving the meal. "When we have finished eating," she said, "I've got some things to share with you . . . and . . . well, I need your advice . . ."

"Anything you say . . . you know that."

After they had eaten and the was table cleared, Carolyn sipped her water and traced designs. Ben noted her weariness . . . started to speak, closed his mouth, and simply waited.

Finally she looked up and smiled wanly. "It's about Dr. Drury," she began, "he . . . he scares me sometimes . . ."

Ben's ire began to rise. "If he so much as . . ."

She touched his arm. "No, Ben. It's not that. It's nothing personal at all . . ."

"Then, what is it?"

"It's the way he dispenses drugs . . . so freely. It's almost as though . . . as though they were harmless . . ."

Her voice shook. "I don't know anyone I can speak to, Ben. But I'm really concerned . . ."

He covered her hands with his and spoke gently. "If you want to talk about it, I'll listen. Okay?"

She drew a deep breath and exhaled. "Okay, I've been holding this in for too long. And, well, to begin, in my opinion, he schedules his patients too close together. Almost back to back, with no time in between. He allows only a few minutes with each of them . . . not enough time to really hear them out . . ."

Ben remembered Anne saying the same thing about Drury. He nodded and she went on.

"He listens for a few minutes, asks a few questions . . . then he reaches for his prescription pad . . . But, that's not the worst of it. Besides the drugs he prescribes, he . . . well, he gives drug samples to everyone."

Withholding judgment, Ben asked, "What about the patients, do they complain?"

"Some of them do. A few of them indicate that they thought their visit with him hadn't been long enough. But they like him. That's just the thing, Ben. Most patients like a doctor like Dr. Drury. He mesmerizes them. He smiles at them, asks about their families, checks their pulses, listens to their hearts. That sort of thing. Then he writes them a prescription and gives them their free drug samples . . ."

"Is it really as bad as all that? I mean, what you're telling me sounds serious, and . . ."

She shook her head emphatically. "Ben, I'm telling you, it *is* serious. It's the overuse of drugs in general, that I'm troubled about, but it's even worse with diet drugs. That scares me. You see, most of our patients are women. And many of them have a weight problem — or think they do. These women generally ask for pills to help them lose weight . . ."

Ben shrugged. "Is that so bad? I mean, diet pills . . . they're not really all that dangerous, are they? Do they have side effects?"

Carolyn was not smiling. "Ben, you've got to realize that drugs are drugs — whether they are prescription drugs or OTC drugs. Over the counter. Because, no matter what kind of drugs they are, all of them have side effects . . . you know who Dr. Arnold Fox is, don't you?"

"You mean the doctor who wrote *The Beverly Hills Medical Diet* a few years ago?"

She nodded. "That's the man. His office is not far from ours. He just published a new book — *Immune for Life*. And in it he makes a very strong statement about drugs. Fox said, 'We doctors act as if we believe that disease is caused by a shortage of prescription drugs in the body.'"[51]

"Coming from a doctor, that's heavy . . ."

"That's not all, Ben. In the same book, Dr. Fox also says, 'I don't know how many patients I've seen who were suffering more from the side effects of their medicines than they were from the original problem.'"[52]

Ben was shaking his head. "Okay, Carolyn, you've made your point. But, diet pills? They're so common . . ."

"Sorry, if I seem to be on a soapbox today," Carolyn said, "but wide usage doesn't mean they're safe. The drugs I'm talking about are advertised every day on TV, and in almost any magazine you pick up . . .

"And, Ben, there are literally *scores* of different brands, all of them with the same dangerous ingredient . . ."

"What ingredient?"

"It's phenylpropanolamine. Difficult to pronounce and spell, and it's used both as a nasal decongestant and an appetite suppressant for weight reduction and control. The information is printed on the container of every product that uses the drug. Most people just don't know . . . and don't read it."

"But the side effects," Ben asked, "what are they?"

"See for yourself . . ."

She picked up a familiar volume, one that Ben had seen Anne use many times. "This is the standby used by all doctors," Carolyn explained, "the *Physicians' Desk Reference*,[53] commonly called the *PDR*. Now, just look at this . . ."

Ben looked. Carolyn was right. In amazement he ran his eyes down the more than one full column of familiar, brand-name products listed under the chemical name of phenylpropanolamine, *in very small print*!

"Here's something else, Ben, a book that every consumer should have in his or her home. It's the *Complete Guide To Prescription & Non-Prescription Drugs*,[54] and it's available in almost any bookstore. It lists over two columns of drugs containing phenylpropanolamine . . ."

Ben was stunned. "Just one more question . . . what are the side effects of this phenylpro . . . something?"

"Glad you asked," she said. "There are lists of them in each of these publications. But here's the brief, two-liner that will make your hair stand on edge. Under the heading of 'Possible Side-Effects' (natural, expected and unavoidable drug actions), it reads: 'Nervousness, insomnia, increase in blood pressure in sensitive individuals.'[55] . . . and that, Ben, is only for starters. From there, it gets worse . . ."

Ben was shaking his head. "That's incredible!"

"What do you mean, incredible?"

"Well, we've been urged to, 'Just say no,' to street drugs, the so-called recreational drugs. Yet, many of the drugs you just showed me can be purchased by anybody in any drugstore. Right?"

"That's true, Ben. So, you can see why I'm so concerned about drugs . . ." She paused.

Ben's head was whirling. But, even above and beyond the drugs they were discussing at the moment, was a question that had bothered him for weeks.

"Carolyn, while you've got all this drug information in front of us . . . let me ask you this — what about the drugs used in cancer chemotherapy — just how dangerous are they?"

Her mouth tensed. "All of them are toxic, some of them extremely so. And some of them are known to be carcinogenic themselves, that is, they actually cause cancer. And, Ben, many times the patient dies from side effects of the drug rather than from the malignancy."[56]

Ben drew a long breath and let it out slowly. He had nothing further to say.

Dr. Anne's Journal

"So, that's it, Ben," Carolyn went on, "and you can see how concerned I am about the drugs that Dr. Drury is giving out . . ."

He had never experienced such pain. It felt like his groin was being ripped apart with a dull knife. When he finally managed to squeeze out a few drops of urine, it was tinged with red. Trembling with fear and pain, Ted stumbled back to bed, each slight move inciting fresh waves of flesh, rending agony.

He was clammy cold, but the effort to pull the sweaty sheets around him reactivated the red-hot poker that was searing his guts with flame . . .

Huddled in a fetal position he felt momentary surcease. Even so, the pressure was still there. He must relieve his bladder, but he feared to move lest he lose consciousness. The groan that wrenched itself from the depths of his being served only to release again the full fury of the demon within.

"Ted . . . Ted, speak to me. Please speak to me." Toni turned on the light. Seeing her husband writhing in agony, she covered her mouth with her hand to withhold a scream.

He heard her voice through the fog of pain and roaring of pain that possessed him. He had to do something . . .

"Toni . . . Toni . . . help me. Please help me!"

"I'll call Dr. Drury . . ." Toni said and moved quickly to the telephone where she had taped Jack's number. Her fingers were trembling . . .

Each faint breath, each stir of finger or toe, reswathed Ted's total being with new intensities of torment . . . wave after wave swept over him, engulfing him, drowning him . . .

After an eternity of eternities, merciful darkness came.

Huntington Memorial Hospital, just twenty minutes from his office, was Jack Drury's hospital of choice, the one to which he instructed the paramedics to deliver Ted Shaffer. The man was in shock when the ambulance arrived, and appropriate action had been taken. Now, pale and drawn, Ted Shaffer was morosely surveying his limited domain when Jack arrived.

Coming directly to the point, Jack said, "Ted, another episode like that and you could be in more trouble than you'd care to consider."

"Yeah, Doctor, I know . . ." He looked away.

"Which means we've got to do something . . ." Jack went on.

Ted sighed deeply. "Yeah, I know that, too . . ." Suddenly he turned back. "But, Doctor, whatever it is, *no surgery*! I mean it. Absolutely no surgery. Understand?"

"Ted, we don't even know what it is . . . so, how . . .?"

"Doctor, I know what it is."

"You can't know — at least for certain, until . . ."

"Okay, Doctor, I'll level with you. I went to Dr. Spicer a month or so ago . . . didn't tell anybody. Not Toni, or anybody. He examined me, took a bunch of tests . . . I've got copies in my briefcase." He paused, seemingly unable to go on.

Jack waited respectfully.

Ted swallowed hard. "And it was what I'd figured all along. Cancer. Prostatic cancer . . . I couldn't tell Toni . . . just couldn't. It'd kill her . . ."

"What did you plan to do?" Jack asked softly.

"I didn't know what to do." He shrugged. "It seemed like the end of the road for me . . ."

"What did Dr. Spicer suggest?"

"He suggested . . . no, Doctor, he strongly suggested, with no other choices, that I be admitted the very next day . . . for surgery. He was going to follow up with chemotherapy . . . maybe radiation

267

. . ." His voice trailed off. "Surgery. Chemotherapy. Radiation . . ." he spoke to nobody in particular.

He roused himself. "Doctor, I'm an engineer. A damned good one. I'm intelligent. And I can read. I'd been reading . . . even before I saw Spicer. I know what the statistics are.

"So . . ." he drew a long, deep breath, grimacing in pain, "so, I said to myself — the route Spicer wanted me to take was a dead end . . ." He chuckled slightly. "No pun intended. So I decided I'd take my chances . . . which I did . . ."

He spread his arms wide, then dropped them in a gesture of hopelessness. "Then I ended up here . . . and I don't know what I'm going to do." He looked up. "Any ideas, Doctor?"

While the man was talking, Jack's mind was whirling, and a bold plan was beginning to form.

He pulled a chair up close to the bed. "Yes, Ted, I *do* have an idea . . . I want you to listen very, very closely . . ."

"You see," Jack began, "you must realize by now, that despite what you may have heard to the contrary, surgery, chemotherapy and radiation, even hormone therapy, do not cure cancer. Nobody can promise a *cure* by any of those modalities. Sometimes some of the damage caused by cancer can be rectified by surgery . . ."

He paused for acknowledgement. Ted nodded his understanding. Ben cleared his throat and went on, "Chemotherapy and radiation do not cure cancer. They merely put it in remission. Or arrest it, slow it down. It's true that chemotherapy and radiation kill cancer cells, but they both do considerable damage to healthy cells in the process.

"And hormone therapy sometimes can help by replacing hormones that the body is no longer able to produce, or that it produces in too small quantities . . . Are you still with me?"

"I'm soaking it all in," Ted said seriously.

"So you see, Ted, " Jack said, "no doctor can cure anybody. Not of cancer. Not of anything. All doctors can do — even at the very best — is help provide a proper atmosphere for the body to do its own healing. Any good doctor will tell you this . . ."

Ted frowned. "Then how can anyone become healthy again?"

"By living healthily . . ."

"It's that simple?"

Jack nodded emphatically. "That simple. And that difficult. Look, Ted, you're an engineer. And a good one. Right?"

"Absolutely. One of the best in my field. But what does that have to do with health?"

"Engineering, per se, nothing. But principles, everything. You see, Ted, most of your work involves mathematics. Causes and effects . . . measurements. Analyses. And so on. Right?"

Ted looked puzzled. "Yes, of course, but I don't see what you're getting at."

"Just this," Jack said, "when you design a building or a structure of any kind, you design it to function according to a plan, don't you?"

"Naturally. But I still don't get it . . ."

"You will. And you design that structure to handle certain stress factors, don't you? *Specific* stress factors . . ."

Ted nodded. "That's right. And I think I see where you're going. If the stress limits are exceeded, then the structure will fail. Is that it?"

Jack chuckled. "That's absolutely correct. Because, to some extent, cancer is not a primary disease. It's partly a reaction to a set of circumstances that weaken the body's defenses. And, Ted, our bodies are built according to a plan. An orderly plan. They are designed to function properly, and if . . ."

"If treated properly," Ted broke in excitedly, "they will do just that. But, if the stress limits are

269

exceeded, parts of the body begin to fail . . . to break down. Right?"

"You've got it," Jack agreed. "Now, let's go a step further. I notice that you drive an Olds . . . an excellent vehicle, and one that requires proper maintenance . . ."

Ted was nodding, beginning to smile.

"And, unless I miss my guess, Ted, you never put junk fuel into that do you? And you always service it according to the manufacturer's recommendations. Am I right?"

Ted was nodding, but he was no longer smiling. "Doctor, I get the picture. I love my car. And I never abuse it. But I have been abusing my body regularly for years . . ."

He absentmindedly traced a pattern on the bed with his finger. Suddenly he looked up. "Doctor, it's becoming clear to me. I'm sick, my health is impaired. Dr. Spicer wants to cut into my body and remove the damaged part. But, I realize, that even if he did successfully remove my abused prostate gland, and cut out all the cancer . . ." he shuddered, "that still wouldn't correct the *cause* of the problem. Right?"

Jack was smiling now. "You're doing fine. I think you can see now, Ted, that the cause of your problem has been abusive living. No doctor can correct that problem. Only you can do that. And I'm not saying that surgery is never necessary, or that it might not be temporarily helpful. But, I don't think that's the real issue here. Right now, your body is talking to you . . . it's begging you for the opportunity to heal itself . . ."

Ted sat up straighter in bed and clasped his fingers behind his head. "Are you telling me that my life depends upon listening to my body . . .?" He grinned weakly at his attempt at humor.

"That's right, Ted. Your life *does* depend upon it."

"Okay, Doctor, beginning right now, I'm listening . . ."

As they were speaking, Toni entered the room. Jack stood up and offered her his chair, moving another one close to the bed for himself. "Please don't let me interrupt you," she said.

"You aren't," Jack told her. "You're just in time . . ."

He turned back to Ted. "With that background, Ted . . . and Toni . . . I'm suggesting that you at least consider a different, perhaps revolutionary therapy . . ."

Ted broke in. "You mean metabolic therapy . . ."

Jack's face reflected the surprise he felt. "What do you know about metabolic therapy?"

Looking for all the world like the cat that ate the mouse, Ted slid a softcover book from beneath his pillow. He held it up with a triumphant gleam in his eyes. "I've been reading this man's story . . ."

"What's the man's name?" Jack asked, attempting to read it on the cover, but Ted was so excited he didn't hold it still.

"Dr. Anthony Sattilaro . . . he's a medical doctor . . ."

Brandishing the book like a baton, Ted said, "He had cancer — and he licked it. He did it through nutrition and metabolic therapy. And if he did it, then I can do it . . ."[57]

Toni looked from her husband to Jack, a look of puzzlement on her face. "I guess I don't quite understand . . . cancer? Metabolic therapy? What are you talking about, Ted? Do you have cancer?"

Jack rummaged in his brief case and held up another book. "To answer your question, Toni, yes, Ted does have cancer. I'm sorry. But, don't panic. I was going to leave this book with you . . . in fact, I will. Among other things, the book lists 25 non-toxic therapies *and* their therapists. Every one of them has a track record of helping people defeat cancer . . ."

He handed the book to Toni. "I suggest you read the whole thing," he said, "but especially Chapter 7 . . . that chapter gives you the names and addresses of 38 real people. *And* their telephone numbers. All of them had cancer — different kinds of cancer — and all of them chose the metabolic therapy route . . ."[58]

"The metabolic route?" Ted said in wonderment. "All of them?"

Jack nodded. "That's right. All of them. But, you don't have to take my word for any of this. You can talk to these people yourself. Ask them to compare cancer statistics — statistics for the surgery, chemotherapy and radiation route — over against the metabolic therapy route.

"These people believe that the survival statistics are on the side of metabolic, or natural therapy. They'll also tell you that the quality as well as the quantity of their lives was and is better during the entire healing process . . ."

Toni suddenly threw her arms around her husband. "Ted . . . Ted . . . we're going to overcome this. I just know it. We're going to win!"

Ted hugged her and held her tightly so she couldn't see the tears that sparkled in his eyes.

Jack quietly left the room.

CHAPTER TWENTY-SIX

By now Ben was amassing a huge stack of notes and a vast store of interviews and information, which he must soon begin shaping into a manuscript. He had gone over Anne's journal so many times that he had committed portions of it to memory. And with each reading he found himself more finely attuned to the complex, tortured psyche he had known as Anne.

Each layer he penetrated enabled Ben to understand her more clearly and to delve more deeply into the cavern of dread and fear in which she had lived . . .

Except for those first few days, he had not worked with Anne's Journal itself, but had made photocopies and placed the original — page markers, loose notes and all — in a safe deposit box. He was glad that he had done so, because on at least one occasion Ben believed that someone had entered his condo, presumably for the purpose of appropriating her journal.

Now, for some reason, he felt frustrated, as though he was missing or overlooking some arcane message that she had intended that he find. Perhaps, he thought, the original will reveal more than the photocopy. So he trekked to the bank and obtained it.

He immediately knew he had been right. Something about the look and feel of that smooth brown leather cover communicated more to him in a moment than had the flimsy photocopy in several months. Stirring up the fire that had died down, Ben settled himself and opened again his wife's journal. He was instantly struck by a truism, how little things, scarcely noticed at the time, suddenly assumed important proportions.

Memories engulfed him . . .

Anne glowed at her wedding.

If mere dollars could have purchased happiness, none could have been happier than she. For it was glitteringly apparent that Collins spent a mint to marry off his daughter. Or, perhaps more accurate, that he expended a mint to make certain that the public was aware of Dr. Anne, and that she was *his* daughter.

But, above all the tintinnabulation, it was clear to all but the most obtuse, that Collins' overriding purpose was to state (or overstate) the fact, that he was a man of political power to be reckoned with. And, corollary to the above, that he had money to spare, and that, at least for this occasion, he was "sparing" it. Lavishly.

For weeks, scores of workmen swarmed over the Peak: painting and polishing, planting, trimming and edging. Restoring it again to its original brilliance. When all was in readiness, a huge tent was erected, caterers and an orchestra engaged, and San Francisco's elite — especially those who dared not snub Collins — gathered to pay homage to their own chthonian deity.

During those last hours of bachelorhood before the big event, Ben wandered freely throughout the mansion. Built around the turn of the century, the Peak was a magnificent edifice of imposing proportions.

The foyer — with imported marble floors, wide, curving staircase of hardwoods no longer available to even the most skilled craftsmen — would have given pause even to a prince. Despite himself, Ben was impressed . . .

He chanced upon what was apparently an informal pre-nuptial reception for a handful of the select that was underway, and slipped unnoticed into a corner to sip an aperitif. At first he was unaware of the male voices quietly engaged in conversation. The subject of their discussion was of no interest to him, so he allowed their words to flow around him without comprehension. Until he heard someone say . . .

". . . she just got her medical degree . . ." He recognized Bert Collins' voice. With a jolt he realized they were talking about Anne. He pricked up his ears.

"Shouldn't make any difference . . ." an unfamiliar voice responded. "Unless she begins asking questions . . ." Someone nearby laughed in a high-pitched voice, and Ben missed a few words . . .

". . . new drug too important for any holistic medicine interference . . . or slip ups . . . if she happened to . . ."

The man dropped his voice and Ben missed the last part of the sentence. Collins laughed harshly and said, "Don't worry, Roger. I'll take care of that . . . I can handle her. I manage to keep an eye on her . . ."

The two men moved away, leaving Ben wondering what it was all about. But in the intense activity that followed, including the thrill of that moment when his radiant bride — her smile for him alone — glided gracefully down the aisle to join him at the altar — the incident slipped from his mind . . .

Startled, Ben reread the journal page, momentarily wondering what had catalyzed the memory of that wedding day incident.

Then he knew. It was that name. Roger. Why had that name stuck in his mind? Perhaps because he'd once gone to school with a boy named Roger.

Dr. Anne's Journal

Anyway, Roger, Roger *somebody* was the man he had
overheard talking with Collins — the two of them
apparently discussing Anne — just before the
wedding ceremony.

In the Journal entry he had just read, one
having to do with the wedding, Anne mentioned the
man's name. Ben read the entry again, very carefully
. . .

> *My wedding day! (Following details
> having to do with the lovely
> arrangements, Anne wrote:) Daddy
> introduced me to Roger Keller. He told
> me Mr. Keller is the chairman of the
> board for Bullion, Inc. International. I
> know he wanted to impress me. But I
> wasn't impressed, even though he told
> me that BII will soon be the biggest
> pharmaceutical company in the
> world. . . .*

"That must have been the man Collins was
talking with that day," Ben mused aloud. "But what
were they talking about . . .?"

As near as he could recall, Ben tried to
reconstruct that conversation. He remembered Keller
being concerned about Anne asking too many
questions. Then he'd mentioned an important new
drug of some kind . . .

He pressed his fingers to his head in
concentration. Then it happened, like a camera lens
snapping into focus, and the picture became clear. He
recalled Collins' exact words: "Don't worry, Roger," he
had said, "I'll take care of that. . . I can handle her. I
can prevent her from embarrassing us . . ."

Dear God, Ben thought, that's what Collins
had done. He had never allowed Anne to slip beyond
his control. He had even placed her in Drury's office,

where he could be informed of her every movement
. . .

He had *ordered* Allen Drury to keep her away
from Jack Drury. He had manipulated and controlled
Anne in every way possible. Why? To protect himself.
To prevent Anne from even thinking about — or in
any way attempting to deviate from — anything
except orthodox ways of practicing medicine.

But there had to be more than that, Ben
knew. Collins must have had an even more
compelling reason than merely Anne's philosophy of
practicing medicine. That, in and of itself, could
certainly not have embarrassed either Collins or BII.
There had to be something more. But, what could it
have been? Why had he been so determined to control
his daughter's future.

The answer to that conundrum must be that
Anne, potentially at least, had had within her power
the ability to embarrass both her father and BII,
probably some power that she herself was not even
aware of. But, what could it have been? Suddenly it
came to him. And he knew . . .

Anne had been a bright, almost brilliant med
student, one apparently destined to perform
independent, original cancer research. Some
professors had encouraged such research and Anne
had longed to pursue that goal. The word had
evidently reached Collins . . . and he had
consequently succeeded in thwarting her plans.

With that awareness, the screen sharpened,
the picture brightened, and Ben had his answer.
Perhaps he could never prove it. But he *knew*.

Even in private practice where he had forced
her, for his daughter to have joined forces with Jack
Drury in asking too many questions about drugs and
drugging, Anne could still have been an
embarrassment to Collins.

Ben reviewed again the puzzling questions she
had agonized over. Questions like: What single entity

controls *all* the cancer research grants? And, Why are grants awarded only to researchers whose efforts lie with the "accepted" guidelines? Why are proven cancer therapies — such as those successfully utilized by scores of therapists and clinics, within and beyond the U.S. — refused "official" sanction?

Scores of such questions, none with answers forthcoming, had frustrated Anne till the very end.

"Yes," he whispered to the empty room, "Anne did have it within her power alone or in cooperation with Jack Drury — to have caused considerable anxiety to the cancer industry, which included BII . . ."

Armed as he now was, with the knowledge of Allen Drury's indirect connection with BII through Collins, and their conspiracy to keep Anne tightly reined, the picture was begining to take shape.

An ugly suspicion forced itself to the forefront of Ben's mind. That day — the day of Phineas' funeral — the time when Anne had gone to her father's office, the time she had revealed to him the fact that she, too, had become a victim of the dread disease, what had been Collins' response . . .?

Ben quickly leafed to that page of her journal. There it was, plain as day. Why hadn't he seen it before? Of course, he knew, it was a basic learning principle: comprehension builds upon comprehension, then all things fall into place . . .

> *Grandfather was buried today . . . (the entry began). I cannot begin to plumb the depths of my loss. Now, as never before, I can fully identify with her. I wonder if she knew or guessed. Afterwards, I went to see Daddy, and in the light of Grandmother's losing battle with cancer through orthodox therapy, to share with him my knowledge of my illness. I don't know exactly what I*

expected, perhaps some sympathy, some
expression of concern. He listened to it
all, unmoved. That is, unmoved until —
based on my growing understanding of
the disease — I began outlining my
projected treatment protocol.
Inexplicably, he became angry, more
angry than I ever remember seeing him.
I am dreadfully confused by it all, but I
am now aware, that for some reason or
reasons unknown to me, my father
would move hell itself to prevent me
from publicly opposing his views . . .

"Then it is true," Ben whispered to the now
dead embers of the fire on the hearth, "it's true, all
that I suspected. Collins sacrificed his daughter, my
wife . . . for monetary gain . . ."

There was not a vindictive bone in Ben's body.
But there were moments, such as the present, when
he longed to pound, to strike out — coldly, viciously
— to maim, to hurt the one who had destroyed his
wife. Overcome with bitterness, he leaped to his feet
and slammed through the door . . .

He roared in angry frustration to the hills.
"Damn you, Collins. Damn you. I pray that you die a
miserable, lonely death. . . and that you roast in the
hell of your own making. Forever. Forever!"

The wind tore the words from his mouth and
slammed them against the hillside where they
reverberated from canyon to canyon. A lonesome
coyote's wail answered him back . . .

Roger Keller was having problems of his own.
Oncoplex had been on the market for two months
now, and the responses had been far beyond what
they had expected. Headlined in newspapers across
the country, followed by feature stories, the media

was touting the miraculous effects of the world's "Newest cancer drug . . ."

> *San Francisco — Bullion's Oncoplex has been proclaimed throughout the City as the cancer miracle drug of the 90s. There seems little doubt that the present one-half million cancer deaths projected for this year will be halved. A wonderful, fantastic miracle!*

Other cities featured similar stories. "Oncoplex is the world's answer to cancer," DJs punned. "Oncoplex removes the hex." The CDC in Atlanta reported "excellent results," and the FDA indicated "our belief in Oncoplex has been justified."

But, when the flow of letters continued, Judine could no longer hide the truth from Keller. Trembling with fear and apprehension, she called for an appointment and laid a stack of them on his desk.

"What's this?"

"Complaints . . . about Oncoplex . . ."

"Complaints? What do you mean?" He indicated a stack of headlines on his desk. "The drug's great . . . we've hit the proverbial jackpot. What do you mean, complaints?"

"Roger, in the past four months, there have been reports of deaths — attributable to Oncoplex . . ."

"You're out of your mind, girl. What're you talking about? I've received no such reports?"

"They've all come to me . . ." she began.

"To you? They should have come to me!" he shouted, now angry and suddenly afraid.

Judine dropped her head. "They came to me. And I . . . I didn't pass them on . . ."

"But, why? I should have been notified . . ."

"At first there were only a handful. From the testing. I thought they were flukes. So I filed them.

Then, when Oncoplex went on the market . . . we've . . . we've gotten a flood of them. At least fifty of them . . ."

"Fifty? Fifty? My God, Judine, do you know what this means?"

She nodded miserably, her voice a mere whisper. "Yes . . . yes, I know . . ."

"It means we've got to pull Oncoplex off the market. It will ruin us . . . it will ruin the company . . ."

Suddenly, he looked with bitter distaste at the craven, broken woman before him. "Who else have you told?" he demanded.

"Nobody. I've told nobody."

"You're sure?"

"Absolutely. Nobody knows except you and I."

More gently now, he spoke soothingly. "Okay, Judine, you're entitled to a well-earned rest. Go home and pack your bags. I'm having arrangements made for you to go and spend some time in the sunshine . . ."

She looked at him in astonishment. "A vacation?"

"Absolutely. You're entitled to it. But," he admonished, "don't breathe a word of this to anybody. Anybody at all. Got that?"

"Yes, I understand. Thanks, Roger. Thanks a lot." Relief written on her face Judine turned and scurried out of his office.

The moment she closed the door, Keller dialed Collins private number, one where he could be reached at any time. It rang twice before Collins picked it up.

"Bert . . . we've got problems. Big problems. I want you in my office tomorrow morning. No later than eight a.m. Okay?"

"Right, Roger. I'll catch the first plane I can get. I'll be there first thing in the morning."

The moment he hung up, Collins called his secretary. "Get me on a plane to New York City. ASAP. I don't care which one it is. Cancel all my appointments tomorrow. You know how to handle them . . ."

Without hesitation, Collins began throwing things into his bag. One hour later he was in the air . . .

"So . . ." Keller summed up, "as it presently stands, that's the situation."

During his machine-gun description of the problem, Keller moved from behind his massive black mahogany desk, where he now braced himself, half sitting, half leaning, nervously swinging an expensively-tooled boot. Bert Collins had sprawled his bulk in one of Keller's black-leather divans. He had bitten off the end of a cigar, but hadn't moved to light it. His full attention was fixed upon Keller.

Keller paused momentarily to catch his breath and Collins began clearing his throat in preparation to respond.

Before he could say a word, Keller said, "Now, Bert, I'm not asking you how we should do it. That's your job. But I'm telling you, BII's got too much invested in Oncoplex to let it go down the drain. Whatever it takes . . . the show is going to go on."

Collins paused with the unlit cigar halfway to his lips. He chuckled mirthlessly. "Roger, they don't call me Old Grizzly for nothing. The show'll go on, I assure you. But it's going to cost you . . . plenty . . ." He demonstrated by rubbing his thumb and fingers together.

Keller shrugged impatiently. "That's a given. As it stands right now, Bullion's got in excess of twenty-five million into Oncoplex . . ."

"With a projected return of that many billion before the patent expires, eh?

"Perhaps. More or less . . . But, the point is, Bert, we've got to get cracking on this. Not today. *Yesterday!*"

Collins flicked his lighter, took several long puffs, then exhaled, allowing a wreath of blue smoke to surround his head. He grinned wolfishly. "Roger, I'm already on the job, A couple of senators and several agency men have, shall we say, pledged their full support?"

He lumbered to his feet. "You'll be interested, I've been doing some house cleaning in California. Got a little action going. You might say it's getting a trifle uncomfortable for our opposition in Los Angeles . . ."

The worry wrinkles on Keller's face relaxed. "Good . . . good. Then I suppose I can consider this little flap over and done with then?"

"Indubitably. It's as good as in the bag."

He was stuffing papers into his huge carry-on case when he paused and looked up. "Oh, by the way, that Kelso woman . . . what about her? How're you going to handle her?"

"Don't concern yourself with her. By now she's out of the country . . . permanently buried in one of BII's research centers. We'll never hear from her again."

Collins hefted his attache case. "Good. Keep sending me copies of all complaints, correspondence . . . everything relating to the Oncoplex campaign. Replenish the PAC fund, the private action fund. I'll be using that rather freely. Same with the campaign fund . . ."

Keller moved toward the door with Collins following.

"Oh, one more thing," Collins said, "a few key people mentioned something about their annual vacation this year . . . I told them to go ahead with their plans . . . assured them we'd take care of the details . . ."

"Right. As usual. I suppose you'll be stopping at the bank before you leave the city?"

"Yeah," Collins said, "I'd appreciate if you'd give them a call. I should be there in about an hour. Tell them I need the usual. Twenties and smaller. No fifties like last time."

The moment the door closed behind Collins, Keller buzzed his secretary. "Call Washington. Get Grant on the line . . ."

He began pacing the office nervously, finally pausing to behold the magnificent view of the Statue of Liberty, the early sun's rays glinting on the Lady's crown. Whatever thoughts that picture brought to mind were cut short by his secretary's voice.

"Mr. Keller. Ready for Mr. Grant."

Keller scooped up the telephone, leaned back in his chair and draped a foot over the corner of his desk. "Hello, Grant. Just met with Collins. He assured me he's taking all necessary precautions . . . he's on top of it. Yeah, you can tell that to your boss. Tell him not to worry . . ."

In the airport limousine, Collins helped himself to a drink. He finished it off and replaced the glass. He hesitated briefly, then picked up the phone and dialed a private number.

"Senator," he began abruptly, "Collins here. Just met with the man. Money's no object . . . whatever it takes. Just stop it. Now! Before any of this gets out. I'll be in Washington this afternoon. I've got everything you asked for. Meet me in my hotel about eight."

Collins loosened his tie and laughed harshly to himself. "With liberty and justice . . . for a few . . ." he paraphrased as he poured himself another drink.

Chapter Twenty-Six

Ted Shaffer was no dummy. He'd known for a long time — at least intellectually — that his lifestyle left a lot to be desired. When Toni and their daughter Betsy had begged him to exercise he would respond, "I don't have time. Anyway, I'm as healthy as a horse . . ."

"At least cut out some of that junk food . . ."

He had laughed at his wife. "But, I don't eat all that much . . . few doughnuts now and then. A few cokes a day. A few cups of coffee . . ."

"And steak a dozen times a week. We both know they're not good for you."

These past three days in the hospital had painfully brought all his wife and daughter's remonstrances to mind. And, along with them, the vivid remembrance of Dr. Spicer's painful examination, and the battery of tests that followed.

A few days after the tests, Spicer's nurse telephoned and requested that he come in. "Doctor Spicer emphasized that he'd like to see you immediately," she said.

The doctor was seated behind his desk studying an opened folder when the nurse ushered Ted in and seated him. Spicer didn't look up immediately, but continued to digest the contents of what was apparently Ted's examination report.

Ted was beginning to fidget when Spicer, without looking up, muttered, "It doesn't look good, Mr. Shaffer . . ."

With that introduction, Ted was tempted to jump up and run from the office. He felt claustrophobic. Trapped. He tried to speak, but words wouldn't come, so he said nothing.

"My initial examination produced some findings that I have now verified . . ." Spicer said, looking up for the first time.

"Palpation of your prostate revealed induration, suggesting prostatic malignancy, which I confirmed by transperineal needle biopsy . . ."

Ted's fear and frustration erupted. "Doctor, I don't know what you're talking about?" he shouted. "Why don't you use words I can understand?"

Voice lowered, but still angry, Ted continued, "I'm an engineer. I'm not stupid. But I get the idea you're trying to snow me with those unpronounceable medical terms. Just give it to me straight. I can take it."

Spicer concealed his anger and chose his words carefully. "I'm sorry, Mr. Shaffer. I'll explain it again . . ."

Ted nodded and consciously relaxed his hold on the arms of his chair. "Thanks . . . please do."

"To put it very plainly, Mr. Shaffer, you've got cancer. Cancer of the prostate. And I . . ."

The word had a devastating effect upon Shaffer. He deflated like a punctured balloon. "Cancer?" He whispered, "Cancer, Doctor? Are you telling me I've got cancer?"

Spicer fiddled nervously with his stethoscope. He spoke softly, almost paternally. "That's right, Mr. Shaffer. Cancer of the prostate. There's no doubt."

The steel band Ted had felt around his chest all the way to the doctor's office contracted. He felt like he couldn't breathe. He gasped. "You're certain?"

"Absolutely. In its late stages . . ."

"Late stages? What . . . what are you saying?"

"We could treat it with radiation therapy. Or surgery. In your case, since the carcinoma is quite advanced, I'd recommend radical retropubic prostatectomy and radiation, and possibly hormone therapy. . ."

Ted growled,"For God's sake, speak English, Doctor. Please! What is this radical retro . . . whatever you just said?"

"Speaking plainly, Mr. Shaffer, I am suggesting the surgical removal of your prostate gland. I further recommend that the surgery be followed with radiation . . . Then, depending upon how you respond, we might follow up with hormone therapy."

Ted gasped. "Surgery and radiation? And hormone therapy?"

"Yes. All of this might be necessary . . ."

"Might be necessary? What does that mean?"

"Since your bone pain suggests that the cancer may have metastasized . . ."

"What do you mean, metastasized?" Ted interjected with heat. "Look, Doctor, I'm not your regular everyday patient. I've already told you that. It's bad enough getting practically a death sentence, without having to try and interpret what you're saying.

"I get the distinct feeling that you can control patients better when you do that . . . I ask you again, give it to me straight. In English . . ."

Spicer responded in anger. His face was flushed and his eyes flashed. "By metastasized, Mr. Shaffer, I mean the cancer has begun to spread . . ."

"Then you're telling me that the cancer has spread to other parts of my body?" Ted challenged.

"To put it simply, the answer is yes."

Ted felt nauseous and angry. Suddenly he arose. "And when do you want to do all of this surgery, and whatever . . ."

Spicer spoke evenly, "I have arranged for you to enter the hospital this evening. And I have scheduled surgery at six a.m. tomorrow morning . . ."

"Doctor, this is too fast. I've got to have time to think. Maybe get a second opinion. To get my head together . . ."

Spicer's voice was cold. "Look, Mr. Shaffer, you came to me. I'm an oncologist. I'm a specialist. You wanted my opinion and I have given it. But, I strongly suggest, that if you want to save your life . . . that you get your affairs in order and admit yourself into the hospital this evening . . ."

Dr. Anne's Journal

Ted had not gone to the hospital. Neither had he returned to Dr. Spicer. He simply, as he admitted to himself, "bit the bullet," ignored the pain and had done nothing. Nothing, that is, until the pain became so intense that he had passed out.

They had taken the catheter out this morning, and he'd had no difficulty since. The thought crossed his mind that maybe he'd go home and forget the whole thing — an idea he knew was crazy and irresponsible. He couldn't deny the fact that he had cancer. But, what was he going to do about it?

Dr. Spicer said that it was bad and had probably spread. Did that mean it was hopeless? Dr. Drury didn't seem to think so. And then there was that Dr. Sattilaro. He had recovered . . .

But, what if he couldn't do what Sattilaro did? Or what if he tried it and it didn't work?

Suddenly depressed, he flipped on the television . . .

At that moment, Toni rushed into the room, bringing with her the wondrous smell of the out of doors. She was breathless as though she'd been running.

"Ted," she gushed, catching her breath, "I read this whole book that Dr. Drury gave us. And it's wonderful. It tells you exactly how to live and how to eat to help your body get rid of cancer . . ."

All at once Ted Shaffer experienced an overwhelming desire to live . . . to take responsibility for his own life . . . and to really go on living . . .

CHAPTER TWENTY-SEVEN

Allen Drury was angry. And scared. Just as he was leaving home to go to his office, Bert Collins had called. "Just thought you'd want to know before it happens . . . the Feds are raiding Jack's clinic this afternoon."

"What? Raiding Jack's clinic?" Allen sat down weakly. "Why? On what charge?"

"They don't need a charge, Al. All they need is a tip. From somebody in the area. That's all they need."

"But who tipped them off?"

Bert purred, "You did, Al. You tipped them off. You told them you had reason to believe they were treating patients with untested, unproven methods . . . and substances . . ."

"But I didn't, Bert. I *didn't*. You know I didn't."

"I know it, Al. And you know it. But *they* don't know it. Just thought you'd like to know about it before it happened."

Without thinking, Allen tossed a couple of yellow capsules into his mouth and swallowed them without water. "My God, Bert, what have you done?"

"You can't say I didn't warn you, Allen. Nothing personal. Just business . . ."

The Santa Ana winds swept across Greater Los Angeles area the entire week, raising

Dr. Anne's Journal

temperatures to an all-time high, making a furnace of
the city's already searing black-top streets and
concrete canyons, adding to the frustration-anger
build-up of a million commuters trapped on the
clogged stop-and-go freeways.

Fortunately Jack Drury and the Shaffers had
gotten an early start, though not quite early enough.
And they had barely passed the Los Angeles
International Airport on the 405 Freeway South when
the traffic suddenly ground to a halt. From there it
was stop-and-go almost all the way to Long Beach.

Jack shook his head. "It gets tiresome, but
there's not much you can do about it . . . "

"Yeah, I know. I've commuted for almost
twenty years now. You just can't outguess it . . ."

After making his decision to go to Mexico, Ted
Shaffer had asked Jack to make the arrangements.
"I'll go you one better," he told them, "I'll drive you
down. If we get an early enough start, I can get you
settled and be back to my office by mid-afternoon."

Before leaving the hospital, Jack called the
clinic in Tijuana. By seven a.m. the following morning
he had picked up Ted and Toni, and they were on
their way. Despite the slow start — and the
unseasonable heat — the day went well. Jack was
back at his clinic by four o'clock . . .

Just thirty minutes before the Federal and
States Attorney marshalls entered the waiting room
and served him with the cease and desist warrant.

"What's this all about?" Jack demanded
angrily.

"We've got our orders . . ." the youngest
marshall said, obviously uncomfortable in the role he
was playing.

"But, what are the charges? I mean . . . you
can't come in here and deprive a man of his living.
Not just like that."

"Sorry, Doctor," said the oldest, "we're only doing our job. You'll have to ask that question of the judge."

"But, when?"

"The order says tomorrow morning. Ten o'clock."

The heat continued throughout the night and into the next day. And, along with hundreds of thousands of other early-rising commuters, Carolyn Kemp found herself trapped in the sweltering freeway traffic . . .

As with most drivers, Carolyn kept her radio tuned to a news station that gave frequent traffic updates. The rest of the time, the radio served mainly as background noise to help distract her from the slow-moving the traffic.

"This is KRFN, your Radio Freeway News . . ." Carolyn's radio droned, "bringing you the local news on LA's hottest morning of the decade . . ." Reaching to turn down the sound, the announcer's next words caught her with hand suspended.

"In today's top story, Dr. Jack Drury, a medical doctor practicing in East Los Angeles, is appealing to the States Attorney's office today, in an effort to restore his right to practice medicine. Yesterday, Dr. Drury said, Federal marshalls served him with an order to refrain from further practice of medicine until or unless he is found innocent of charges.

"Apparently the charges stemmed from Drury's releasing a cancer patient from a local hospital and transporting him across the border into Tijuana, Mexico. Mr. Shaffer, Dr. Drury said, had refused surgery and radiation and had chosen to admit himself to a Tijuana cancer clinic. However, Dr. Richard Spicer inferred that Dr. Drury had influenced Shaffer to ignore the results of his tests which indicated the necessity of immediate surgery and radiation to save his life. The States Attorney's office refused to comment. At the moment, no trial date has been set. . . .

"In other local news, a fire broke out in . . ."

"Oh, no!" Carolyn exclaimed in disbelief. "Not Jack . . .!"

She turned off the radio and drove in silence. How can they do that to him? The patient made the decision, not Jack. Maybe I'm getting paranoid, she thought, but it *does* seem like somebody's out to get Jack. And maybe the rest of us.

Two minutes later she merged right and took the Sunset Boulevard offramp to Dr. Allen Drury's Beverly Hills office. Her phone was ringing as she unlocked her door. It was Jack. He sounded grim. "Have you heard the news . . .?" he began.

"Yes," Carolyn interrupted, "on the freeway news. Oh, Jack, what happened?"

"I can't tell you much right now," he said tersely. "Maybe this evening. Will you do me a favor and call Ben? I think he needs to hear the story . . . uh, and tell my father . . ."

"Yes, Jack. Your father just came in. I'll tell them both. And, Jack . . .?" She paused. What was there to say?

"Yes? Yes, Carolyn . . .?"

"Please take care . . . and stay in touch. Okay?"

"Thanks. I'll try." He hung up first.

The telephone still in her hand, Carolyn hesitated. Taking a deep breath, she cradled the phone and walked to Drury's office. She rapped and he looked up. His eyes were puffy, with dark circles around them. He didn't smile. "Yes, Carolyn . . .?"

"It's about Jack . . ." she began. "He called and left a message . . ." As simply as possible, she related Jack's words. Drury gasped and sat down slowly, clutching his chest.

"Dr. Drury!" Carolyn shouted, starting around his desk. "May I get you something?"

He shook his head. "No . . . no, thanks. I'll be all right."

As she hesitated, Drury seemed to regain his aplomb. He spoke again, this time quite harshly. "I said, *I'll be all right*! Close the door on your way out . . ."

Back at her desk, Carolyn realized she was trembling. She sat down and drew a few deep breaths before picking up the phone. She knew Ben had worked late the night before and might still be sleeping. She dialed his number.

He was swimming in the surf on a dark shore, suddenly caught by a strong undertow. The swift, vicious tide was forcing him out to sea and the shoreline was receding rapidly. He tried to strike out toward land, but was hindered by the huge masses of kelp that were entangling his feet and legs . . .

The harder he fought, the more tightly the slippery seaweed wrapped around his legs. As he tried to scream, he was sucked beneath the waves, and his mouth and lungs gulped in huge drafts of salty water.

Inexplicably he popped to the surface, the seas calmed, and he found himself — still enmeshed in the kelp's clammy tentacles — cast upon a familiar Malibu beach. Somewhere near at hand a telephone was ringing.

Telephone? on the beach?

It rang incessantly, insistently. He opened his eyes. Bright sunlight was streaming through his partially drawn drapes. His legs were tightly bound by his damp, twisted sheets . . .

The telephone . . .

He fumbled and picked up the instrument. "Hello . . ."

"Hi, this is Carolyn . . ."

"Uh, good morning."

"Ben. Sorry to wake you. Look, I can't talk long. I'm at the office. I just got a call from Jack . . . he's in trouble . . ."

Ben jerked himself loose from the clinging sheets. "Trouble! What kind of trouble?"

"His clinic was raided last evening. He asked me to call and let you know. Call me when you can . . ."

"Wait. Wait, Carolyn. Raided? What for?"

"That's all he told me . . ."

Ben's fingers on the phone felt slippery with sweat. "Does his father know yet?"

Her voice was muffled like she had suddenly clamped her hand around her mouth. "Yes. I just told him. I thought he was going to have a coronary. He's in his office now. On the phone. I don't know who he's talking to. Look, Ben, I've got to go. Bye . . ."

Ben shook his head to clear it of the nightmares — both the dream and the reality. What to do? Ah, Jack. He quickly punched the numbers, listening impatiently as the phone rang a dozen times before it was picked up.

A rough voice yelled, "Yes, what do you want?"

"May I talk to Dr. Drury?"

"Hold on. I'll see." He heard scrambled bits of a shouted conversation. Then, "Yeah. Hold on. He'll be here in a minute."

It was a long minute. Finally, Jack's strained voice said, "Hello . . ."

"Jack, this is Ben. Carolyn called me. Said you wanted me to know . . . What can I . . .?"

"Nothing. Nothing. Thanks for calling, Ben. But don't get mixed up in this. Talk to you later . . ." The phone clicked. Ben hung up slowly.

Fully awake now, Ben thought a moment, ran his fingers through his hair, then dialed. "Good morning, doctor's office. Carolyn speaking . . ."

Chapter Twenty-Seven

"Hi. Ben. Can you talk?"

"One moment. I'll put you on hold. I have another call." Carrying his portable phone, Ben walked into the bathroom and began shaving. He was halfway through before he heard, "Hi, Ben. I can talk now. But not for long. How's Jack?"

"I don't know. He was very guarded. Probably couldn't say anything . . ."

"What do you think?" she asked.

"I don't know. Did he tell you what his father told him?"

"About the possibility of losing his medical license?"

"Yes," Ben said. "It sounds like somebody, I can't imagine who, turned him in . . ."

"But, what for?"

"Can't tell you, Carolyn. Probably trumped up charges of some kind. Anyway, can you come to my place after work? I'll try and reach Jack to see if he can meet us there . . ."

"Sure. About six-thirty. See you then. Gotta go. Bye."

Ben stripped the sweaty bed and made it up with clean sheets. He tossed the bedclothes into the washer before he got in the shower. By the time he finished it was nearly noon. He tried to reach Jack a couple of times, but there was no answer, and no answering device.

Scratching his head in concentration, Ben paced the length of his living room for half an hour, then dropped in the chair and dialed Hannibal's private number. "Ross, Ben Rush here. I've got a question for you?"

"Give it to me."

"Does Cutting Edge have a good attorney?"

"The very best," Hannibal said. "Why? Got a problem?"

"No, but Jack Drury might. You remember me speaking of him?"

"Sure, the young doctor. What kind of a problem?"

Ben hesitated. "Well, I don't know much yet. But apparently he was raided this morning. I mean, his clinic?"

"Raided? Any idea why?"

"Not really. Just . . . well, his father told him last week he'd better keep away from alternative practitioners. Suggested that somebody might be out to get him . . . then this. Not much to go on. But, that's all I know . . ."

Hannibal was silent for a long moment, thinking. Then he said, "Ben, you sound kinda worried yourself. You sure that's all you've got to tell me?"

Ben drew a deep breath. "Well, there is something else . . . I've been out of town a couple of days. San Diego and Tijuana. Research. When I got back to my condo late last night I knew somebody had been in here . . ."

"Anything missing?"

"Not that I could tell."

"The journal," Ross said. "I think somebody was looking for Anne's journal."

"I agree."

"Looks to me like you're getting into somebody's hair, and they don't like it," Ross said. "Do you still want to keep going on the project?"

"More than ever, Ross. More than ever."

"Thanks, I'll give the attorney a call. He'll get back to you this afternoon . . ."

"Should I call the police and report the prowler?" Ben asked.

"Let's ask Connell. That's the attorney. See what he has to say about it. Okay?"

"Fine, Ross. Thanks. I'll keep you posted."

Chapter Twenty-Seven

That afternoon Ben made a quick trip to Radio
Shack for a couple of items, then stopped by the
Santa Monica Library. He scanned the computer
index, jotted down a few book titles and asked for
them at the reference desk. An hour later, after
photocopying several pages, he returned the books.

By then it was mid-afternoon. Just time to
stop by Gelson's in Marina Del Rey for some fresh
produce. At home again, he tried Jack's number with
no success. Connell, Ross's attorney had called and
left a message. Ben returned the call, asked a few
questions and thanked him. He checked the time.
Five-fifteen. Just time to get a meal together for the
evening . . .

"Carolyn, I think Pauling's onto something,"
Ben was saying. "Among other things, he believes
you've got to enhance cancer patients' immune
systems . . . because the immune system plays an
important role in general cancer treatment . . ."

"Ben, I'm sorry," Carolyn said, "please forgive
me. I am interested in what you're telling me . . .
but, not now. Not knowing about Jack . . . I, I just
can't concentrate . . ."

Ben stopped his pacing and stood in front of
her. "To tell you the truth, I can't either. It's just
that I thought I had to say something or go crazy."

When Carolyn stopped by after work, Ben had
a bowl of fruit and a plate of nut breads ready to eat.
The two of them had taken a few bites, but found out
they weren't hungry. Ben tried to fill the empty time
by sharing some of his newly-acquired research
having to do with Linus Pauling.

But . . . it was no use . . .

"If only he would call," Carolyn began.

Just then the doorbell chimes rang. Ben strode
to the door and Jack staggered in, his clothes
rumpled, hair tousled, looking like he'd spent the day
in the county jail.

Dr. Anne's Journal

"Hi," he said wearily, "got something to eat?"

Then they were all talking at once.

"Hold it, hold it," Jack said. "Let me catch my breath. I've got a story to tell you that you'll find hard to believe . . ."

Ben grabbed him by the shoulders. "Jack, before you do anything, why don't you take a long, hot shower, put on some clean clothes . . . and then we'll hear your story . . ."

Jack allowed himself to be pushed into the bathroom. A few moments later they heard him singing.

"It was just like a James Bond thriller," he was saying. "I had just gotten inside the office. Earl was already there. Maria was coming in the door . . . and whoosh! There they were . . ."

"Who were there?" Carolyn shouted. "Who . . .?"

"The cops. About a dozen of them. With guns drawn. Police dogs on leashes. Flak suits and helmets. Bullhorns . . . the whole bit . . ." He paused, and grinned wryly. "At least they did it up right, Hollywood style."

"Did they have legal papers?" Ben asked.

"Yep. They did it right. At least legal. By the book."

"What did they want?" Ben demanded. "What were they looking for? Anything in particular?"

"Yep. Somebody had reported us as having treated patients with — get this — with unproven substances . . ."

Jack chewed and swallowed a huge mouthful. "They took all our records, files, patient records, everything out of our store room . . . cleaned out the place. Then they took me down to City Hall . . ."

Ben was silent for a thoughtful moment, then asked softly. "Do you have any idea who made out the complaint?"

Jack nodded. "Yep. They showed it to me . . ."

"Who was it?"

Jack had a strange look upon his face. "The signaturé was Allen Drury, M.D."

"What?" Carolyn shrieked. "Your own father?"

Jack nodded. "That's what the signature said. But . . . he didn't do it . . ."

"Didn't do it?" Ben said. "How do you know?"

For the first time Jack laughed. "Look, do you have any idea how many times I've seen my father sign a prescription? That wasn't any more his signature than it was the president's."

CHAPTER TWENTY-EIGHT

It seemed to Ben that he had always been interested in sports and physical fitness. Tennis, swimming and surfing had captured his interest from the time he was small, as it had the majority of his friends. Since college, his increasingly heavy writing schedule made the indulgence in such sports rather inconvenient, which meant he had to seek other ways to provide his body with the necessary exercise.

In Santa Monica, he jogged along San Vicente Boulevard or the beach four or five mornings a week. During his times at the cabin — more frequent and of longer duration — he often shoved a lunch in his backpack and hiked the rugged hills. Those hiking forays, along with his daily half-mile walk down the steep driveway to the mailbox, then up again, provided him with all the cardio-vascular activity he needed.

In addition, he frequently greeted the sunrise by splitting the huge stack of wood he managed to burn in his fireplace each evening as he went over the computer printouts of his daily writing output.

Saturday morning, as he paused to wipe sweat from his eyes, he heard the high-pitched whine of a car making its way up the steep hill. As he watched, he caught a glimpse of a bright green vehicle nosing around a hairpin bend . . .

Dr. Anne's Journal

Carolyn Kemp, an only child, had been loved, cuddled and indulged by her prominent oncologist father, Stephen Kemp and mostly ignored by Bev, his socially-prominent wife. Nevertheless, aside from her frightening episode with polio as a child, Carolyn had become a surprisingly normal teenager.

Because she loved and emulated her father, it seemed only natural to make medicine her career choice; but a nurse instead of a doctor. "Why nursing?" Kemp asked when she announced her decision, "and not a full-fledged medical professional?"

"Father, I happen to believe that a nurse *is* a full-fledged medical professional. And, as far as becoming a doctor, I don't want all the hassles and responsibilities . . ."

Beverly simply sniffed haughtily. "Carolyn, *dahling,* why *become* anything? Why not just bag some oil-rich Arab or wealthy Beverly Hills type?"

"Mother! I don't want to bag anybody. I want to be myself. If a man wants me, let him try to *bag* me . . ." Carolyn refrained from adding what she was thinking, Besides, Mother, you and most of that TV crowd you speak of, party too much to suit me.

Beverly kept herself bean-pole thin by her chain smoking. Both her husband and daughter deplored the vice, but knew Bev well enough to say nothing.

As for her own figure, Carolyn admitted that she was a bit overweight, but rationalized, "as long as I am healthy . . ." It was because of Jack Drury's influence that she became more selective in her eating habits.

Carolyn lived at home until she graduated and earned her R.N. cap. She announced her independence by investing a portion of the trust fund she'd inherited from her grandfather's will, and purchased a condo in Marina Del Rey. Refusing her father's offer to work in his office, at her mother's suggestion, Carolyn interviewed for and accepted the opening in Allen Drury's office, Bev's personal physician.

Most men bored her, so she dated infrequently. And not until she met Jack Drury had she met a man who challenged her mind. Now, with the advent of Ben Rush, who excited her like no one else she had ever known, she found herself with two possibles. What should she do?

All these thoughts had been running through her mind for days. Except for that moment when Ben had kissed her, neither of the men had made a move in her direction. Perhaps, she thought, it was time for her to initiate a move of her own . . .

For the first time in years, Carolyn felt restless and unsettled. And lonesome . . .

What about Ben?

Should she call him? Make a date with him for the day? Then she remembered . . . he wasn't in Santa Monica. He'd told her and Jack that he was going to his cabin that night.

Then, she reasoned, why not invite herself out there? She was familiar with Malibu and Ben had once verbally sketched out his cabin's locale. Yes, she decided, the idea had merit.

With school-girl anticipation, feeling suddenly adventurous, she bolted upright in bed. "Yes, that's what I'll do," she said aloud. "I'll surprise him."

She checked the clock. It was five-fifteen and dark outside. Within minutes she had showered, dressed and was headed toward Malibu in her bright green Alpha Romeo. She felt more carefree and euphoric than she'd felt for ages . . .

Ben didn't try to disguise his pleasure. He dropped his ax and welcomed her with a hug. Despite herself, Carolyn felt the blood rush to her cheeks.

"Welcome to my Hawk's Hangout," he said with an expansive gesture.

"Hawk's Hangout? I've never heard you use the term before."

"Because I never did before. It just came to me," he laughed. "And I do have lots of hawks cruising the area . . ."

Within minutes they were preparing breakfast: a huge one, because they were both hungry. Afterwards, they settled in front of the native-stone fireplace and sipped their hot herbal tea. Suddenly shy, Carolyn ventured, "Ben, I really should have called . . . shouldn't I?"

His exuberant chuckled echoed in the large room. "Why should you have called? I haven't done anything but work for months. Your coming gives me an authentic reason for being lazy . . ."

Dressed in faded jeans, flannel shirt and worn boots, she thought he looked more like a rancher than a writer. His skin and eyes glowed with health. In keeping with the spontaneity of her mood, she had also slipped into a pair of jeans, and had chosen a hot pink top to accentuate her platinum hair. Looking up suddenly, she caught his frankly approving glance.

Now that I'm here, she thought, what do I do?

She settled on a question. "Ben, doesn't it seem a little bit unusual for a doctor like Jack to be raided? I mean, it seemed to me they were treating him as a common criminal."

"Actually, Carolyn, from what I've been learning . . . what happened to Jack is not an isolated incident . . ."

His reply surprised her. "Do you mean that . . .?"

He nodded. "In these past few weeks of networking . . . research for the new book, you know . . ."

She nodded in the affirmative. "What's your major focus?"

Chapter Twenty-Eight

A shadow of pain crossed his face. "Cancer," he said simply. "Alternative methods of treating patients with cancer . . ."

"Because of Anne?"

"It started that way. But now the whole project's taken on a life of its own." The morning was chilly so Ben arose and tossed more wood on the fire.

"Anyway, to answer your question. I've come across quite a number of health practitioners who have had difficulties with what I now recognize as the Cancer Establishment. I've gotten to know some of these people . . . some have gone to jail. Others have lost their hospital privileges. And quite a few have had their medical licenses revoked . . ."

"But, why? I don't understand . . ."

For an hour Ben outlined the information he had unearthed.

"Basically, or you might say, the bottom line is this: The ones who have gotten into trouble are the ones who dared to begin questioning in ways that run contrary to the orthodox way of doing things . . ."

She interrupted with a sudden thought, horrifying in its implications. "Ben? Do you think Anne was becoming a threat?"

His lips tightened. "I don't know for sure. I'm still digging . . ."

To cover the emotions that expressed themselves on his face, Ben turned and poked the fire. When it blazed brightly, he sat down again, his hands clenched tightly between his knees. To hide their trembling, Carolyn thought.

"The questioners' problems manifest in a number of different ways — all for a single purpose: to intimidate, and by so doing, to force the errant ones back into line . . ."

"Like raiding them . . . such as they did with Jack?"

He shrugged. "Sometimes. Not always. It depends. Depends on how flagrant the so-called deviations from orthodoxy. The harassment — for that's precisely what it is — may begin with a raid. That's a warning . . .

"If the recalcitrants don't heed the warning, they might find themselves in court, for months. Sometimes years. It's a Catch-22 situation. No-win. After a long court battle, they may win the battle. That is, the judge *might* possibly rule in the deviator's favor. It does happen. Not often, but it does. Even then, to their chagrin, 'winners' quickly learn that even though they won the battle, they've lost the war . . ."

Carolyn nodded, comprehension dawning. "You mean, loss of credibility *and* patients . . ."

"Yes, and sometimes temporary loss of license to practice. Occasionally this loss is for only months or a year or two. But I have personally met two — and know of a number of others — where this loss is permanent."

"You can't be serious!"

"I am serious. Very serious. But, that's only part of the story. Even though they managed to keep their license, the long, drawn out legal battle may have exhausted all their financial resources, so they end up broken. Business down the drain. Often with nothing to show for a lifetime of work . . ."

Carolyn's face was pale with emotion. "That's horrible. It's unspeakable. Terrible!"

His grin was grim. "No doubt about it."

Ben's expression softened. "Carolyn, I'm sorry to . . . well, to apprise you of this damned situation . . ." He shrugged. "But I thought . . . well, since you were involved, at least indirectly, that this background information might give you a clearer picture of what's happening . . ."

She nodded, but didn't respond immediately. For a long moment they both stared meditatively into the glowing embers on the hearth. When she began speaking, it was evident that she had given much thought to the words she was saying.

"Ben I know that Dr. Allen Drury is in some way implicated in the situation . . ."

He was surprised. "What do you know? I mean, how much do you know about Allen Drury?"

"Some things I know . . . some things I suspect. But I know for a fact that Mr. Collins has some power over Allen . . ."

Ben nodded. "I want to hear about that. But, I'd like some more tea. How about you?"

"Yes, please."

From the kitchen, Ben asked, "A little more lemon?"

"Yes. I use quite a bit of lemon."

Seating himself, Ben said, "I think you might be onto some information I need. What kind of power does Collins hold over your boss? And, how do you know?"

Carolyn absentmindedly stirred and tasted her tea. "For several years now, Dr. Drury has had me open all the mail, even the letters marked personal. The bills I pay . . . of course, Dr. Drury signs all the checks. I just get them ready for him . . ."

She looked up and Ben nodded.

"Also, I handle all of the incoming telephone calls. As well as some of the outgoing calls. Sometimes Dr. Drury will have me get some people on the line before he takes them . . ."

"Saves him quite a bit of time," Ben commented.

"Of course. He needs that. He's a very busy doctor." She paused to sip her tea. She looked directly at Ben. "Do you know anything about BII?"

"You mean Bullion, Inc., International? Yes, a little. Why?"

"Did you know that they just launched a multi-million dollar advertising campaign for their new cancer drug, Oncoplex?"

He nodded his head. "I read something about it in *The Times*. Sounds like it might make them a bundle of money. Why do you ask? Does Drury have something to do with BII?"

She nodded. "Dr. Drury has *a lot* to do with BII. A lot of dollars. He invested over $100,000 in Oncoplex. I know. I opened the correspondence . . ."

Ben whistled. "That's a *lot* of somethings to do with BII."

"But, there's more. My father is an oncologist, a cancer specialist. I asked him what he knows about Oncoplex. He gets all the literature on new drug releases. He told me that BII is touting it as the 'cancer drug of the century' . . ."

"What does Dr. Kemp think of Oncoplex?"

"He's viewing it with caution. He's heard rumblings about there being some problems with it. Some serious problems — fatalities . . ."

"Okay, I get all this, but, Carolyn, how does it all tie together? I mean, Dr. Drury? Bert Collins? BII?"

Carolyn got up and stretched, then began to pace nervously as she talked. "I was coming to that. About a week ago Dr. Drury got a personal letter from Roger Keller. He's BII's Chairman of the Board and CEO. I suppose all their big investors received the same letter . . ." She paused for breath.

"Most likely," Ben commented.

"Here's the thing that really caught my eye, Ben. Among other things, Keller encouraged the recipients to do everything they could to discourage unorthodox cancer modalities — *with all the means at their disposal.*"

"Then, that begins to explain why Allen tried to shy Jack away from his divergent interests . . ."

Carolyn paused in her pacing. "Yes, but there's something else that bothers me. You knew, of course, that Bert Collins' legal firm handles all or most of BII's legal work?"

Chapter Twenty-Eight

His mouth open to speak, Ben jumped up . . .

She held up her hand. "Just a minute. There's more . . ." She gave him an imploring look. "Ben, I would have told you all this, but it didn't all come together until they raided Jack. Then I knew there had to be some tie ins . . ."

"And there are. Are there ever!"

"Well, here's the clincher. Allen Drury and Bert Collins have known each other for a long time. For a long, long time. And, before they went to Stanford . . . you knew that they went there together, didn't you?"

Ben nodded.

"Anyway, I happened to overhear a telephone conversation between Dr. Drury and Collins one day. Collins said, 'You owe me one,' and Dr. Drury acknowledged it. Then he said something I didn't understand then, and still don't . . ."

She stopped and Ben noticed how pale her face had become.

"Carolyn, is something wrong?"

She drew a deep breath and shook her head. "Well . . . yes. Actually there is. There was this phone call that took place before I knew you. It didn't seem significant at the time . . ." Her voice sounded tired and strained.

He looked puzzled. "What do you mean?"

"Well, Collins was telling Dr. Drury to keep Jack away from the alternative care clinics . . . *and his daughter* . . ."

Ben drew his breath in sharply. From the beginning, the nagging thought had plagued him that in some way Collins had been behind Anne's refusal to accept anything but orthodox modalities to treat her cancer.

Even though *she'd apparently known* all along that such a decision might cost her life . . .

CHAPTER TWENTY-NINE

Following this past Saturday with Ben, Carolyn found herself more and more drawn to the man. His singlemindedness impressed her, as did his ability to assimilate and synthesize masses of eclectic information and form it into a cohesive whole. She had no doubt that he liked her. But she also had the distinct feeling that unless or until he cleared up the troubling circumstances surrounding Anne's choice of cancer treatment, Ben would be invulnerable to her as a woman.

"If that's the case," she spoke aloud in her car as she pulled onto the North 405 onramp and moved into the fast lane, "I'll do everything I can to help him."

Allen Drury was late returning to the office from his hospital rounds, and several patients were already waiting for him when he arrived. He seemed to be nervous and jittery and gave the appearance of not having slept well or long enough.

He was uncharacteristically rude to her on two occasions when she had merely handed him the information he had requested minutes before. Neither time had he seemed to be aware of either his words or his attitude. His patients also noticed Drury's preoccupation and several of them mentioned it to her.

All in all, she was thankful when the last patient had gone and it was time to close the office.

Dr. Anne's Journal

As she gathered her things in preparation for leaving, Drury stopped by her desk. "Come into my office, please," he said abruptly, and without waiting for her response, turned and strode down the hall.

Seated now in his office, she tried not to appear as tense as she felt. They had been so busy all afternoon that she hadn't had time to observe him closely. Now, seeing him up close, she was appalled at his drawn and haggard appearance. His eyes were muddy-brown, the pupils dilated. She couldn't bear to look into them and slid her gaze beyond him, to the slightly opened cabinet behind his shoulder. She gasped . . .

He came bluntly to the point. "How much did Jack tell you?"

With an effort she pulled her eyes away from the cabinet to answer him. "He . . . he just told me he'd been raided . . . by the authorities . . ."

That Drury was under tremendous emotional stress was clear. Subliminally, Carolyn noted his rapid and shallow respiration. As well as his pulse rate — easily counted from force of habit by observing his throbbing carotid artery — which was much too fast. Drury's face was flushed and he seemed peculiarly unaware of the way his hands fluttered nervously.

"Nothing else?" Drury demanded in a voice that was at the same time hoarse and harsh.

More alarmed by the man's appearance than by his attitude, Carolyn hesitated. "Doctor . . . are you . . . are you unwell?"

"Of course I'm not unwell. I'm a doctor. Remember?" There was a harsh edge to his voice.

"Now, Miss Kemp . . . what else did Jack tell you?" Drury hadn't addressed her so formally since the first month she worked with him. Something was terribly, terribly wrong.

"Well . . . he spoke of being taken down to the police station . . . and . . ."

"Did he tell you that I had signed the complaint? Did he?"

"Yes . . ."

"He told you that!"

"Yes, Doctor, but he . . ."

But Drury was no longer listening. Drury gasped for breath and slumped across his desk . . .

His head down, hands stuffed in his pockets, Jack Drury nervously paced the gleaming hallways of Cedars-Sinai Hospital. How ironical, he thought, Dad has attended to hundreds of patients in these rooms. Now he has joined them in their pain and suffering. And I — having shared good news and bad with the families of some of those patients — am now as one of them: uncertain, fearful. Waiting . . .

Carolyn still wore her white uniform and crepe-soled shoes, which made no noise as she approached Jack in the corridor. He was unaware of her presence until she spoke . . .

"Jack . . ."

He jerked his head up. "Oh, Carolyn. Thank God you've come."

She smiled. "How could I not come? How is he?"

He shook his head. "You know the reports. 'As well as can be expected. We're doing all we can do.' . . ."

"Yes, but . . . how *is* he?"

"I don't know. I haven't seen him yet. He's in ICU." He took her gently by the elbow. "Let's go to the cafeteria . . . where we can talk . . ."

Neither of them was hungry, so they took a corner table where they wouldn't be disturbed. "Tell me everything . . . tell me exactly what happened . . ."

She related the incident, ending with, "He'd apparently been stressed out all day . . . patients even noticed it. Then, when he began talking about you . . . well, it was just a bit more than he could handle. That's all I know."

"What do you think?" He asked. "CVA, a stroke?"

She smiled slightly. "Jack, I'm a nurse. *You're* the doctor. I can't diagnose. You know that."

He nodded impatiently. "C'mon, Carolyn. I know all that. I also know you're one of the best. Now, tell me, do you think it was a stroke . . . or . . ."

She tilted her head and looked at him. "Jack, I honestly don't know. It could have been a stroke. Heart, maybe. Or, it might have been . . ." She paused, a question in her eyes.

"Might have been *what*? Drug reaction? Is that what you're trying to tell me?"

A stricken look in her eyes, she nodded.

He covered her hand with his. "Carolyn, you don't have to protect him from me. Or feel that you've betrayed him. I knew about the drugs. Even Ben knew. He told me . . ."

She uttered a sigh of relief. "I'm glad, Jack. Not about the drugs. But that you knew. You see, after the ambulance came and took him . . . and before I called you and came over here . . . well, I checked the cabinet in his office . . ."

"And?"

"Jack, it was stuffed, I mean *stuffed* with drug samples. Stimulants and depressants. And narcotics. All kinds of them. And all of them from BII . . ."

"What did you do with them?"

She shook her head. "Nothing. I didn't know what to do. If anything's done, you'll have to do it."

Ben was still at his computer when she called. "Ben, I know it's late . . . but I'd like to come over. May I?"

"You sound . . ."

"Frightened? Confused?"

"Well, yes . . . or . . ."

"Lonesome?" she asked with a slight, nervous laugh.

"That, too. Are you? Any of those?"

"All of the above . . ."

"Is there anything in particular?"

"Yes, Ben. Dr. Drury's in the hospital. Possible stroke. Heart attack, maybe. Might even be a drug reaction. I'd like to talk . . ."

"I'll be waiting for you . . ."

She looked so wan and desolate when Ben answered the door that he reflexively opened his arms and enfolded her. To his surprise, she was sobbing. He held her till she ceased trembling, then seated her in the huge rocker in front of his small, but cheerfully, comforting fireplace.

Without a word, he tucked a blanket around her shoulders, then removed her shoes and massaged her feet. When they had warmed somewhat, he slipped on a pair of wooly slippers.

Her large eyes followed him as he went into the kitchen for the already prepared tea tray and hot, buttered toast. "It was too much all at once . . ." she began, a slight quaver in her voice. "And I didn't know anywhere else to go . . ."

"Where else?" he smiled. "The tea will warm you. Drink it."

She sipped the tea and nibbled at the toast. "Jack is . . .?"

She nodded. "Yes . . . at the hospital. I left him there."

"Had he seen his father yet?"

"Not when I left. He was very upset."

They fell silent, gazing into the glowing embers. After a while he asked, "Do you want to talk about it?"

She smiled for the first time. "Yes, I think so . . ."

Dr. Anne's Journal

Carolyn told him then, about the day — Allen's brusqueness, his rudeness, followed by his interrogation. And the climax. She shuddered, "When . . . when he just fell over on the desk. On his face. I was terrified . . ."

She pulled the blanket tightly around her shoulders. "I shouldn't have been so frightened, should I? I'm a nurse . . ."

He chuckled. "Even nurses — doctors, too — are human. Why shouldn't you have been upset. It was so totally unexpected."

She had called the paramedics and the hospital. "They came so quickly. Only five minutes or so. But it seemed like a long, long eternity. While I was waiting for them, I called Jack . . ."

She hesitated. "Ben . . . before all that . . . I mean, when Dr. Drury and I were sitting there in his office, well, I was facing his cabinet behind him — the door was partially open. And I saw . . . oh, God, I wish I hadn't seen . . ."

"Hadn't seen what?"

"The drugs, Ben. The drugs. I could see them all the while he was talking. I could hardly take my eyes off them to respond to him. And after I called the ambulance and Jack, I opened the doors and looked inside . . ."

She drew a deep breath and released it slowly. "And, Ben, the cabinet was literally filled with drugs. Prescription drugs! Drugs and narcotics. And all of them from BII . . ."

As often as he had seen patients in the intensive care ward, Jack Drury had never become accustomed to the ICU ambience. "What the desperately ill patient needs," he once remarked to a staff physician, "is peace and quiet. But the ICU is anything but peaceful . . ."

The man had looked at Jack sharply, then responded, "You're right, of course. Yes, I know, it's a paradox. But there doesn't seem to be much we can do about it."

"The price of progress?"

"Something like that."

Now, seeing his father wired, tubed, taped and otherwise attached to a roomful of sophisticated electronic, state-of-the-art robotic gadgetry that dripped, printed, hummed, clicked or buzzed in a weird cacophony of confusion as they monitored his vital signs, Jack wondered about the "personal touch" that was once so important to medicine.

Even the harried-looking, overworked nurses supervising this Orwellian nightmare put him in mind of an ant hill with workers scurrying back and forth, each intent upon his or her individual task, seemingly unaware of all else.

"Five minutes. No more," the supervisor told him.

Looking down upon his father, Jack caught his breath. How old, how *diminished* he appeared. It wasn't right or proper for him to be lying here so passively. With a jolt he realized: my father's not a doctor now. He's a patient. And as a patient, he's not in charge anymore, of his body or his mind. Or anything.

Hospital-administered drugs controlled his mind; machines controlled his body . . . an iatrogenic *detenu* . . .

Jack shuddered.

As every patient must do in a like situation, his father had released himself into the hands and ministrations of the medical establishment. And they had transformed him from a man into a patient . . .

Allen Drury's eyes were open, but they were expressionless, dull and uncomprehending. Jack picked up his father's hand. It was dry and cold. And nerveless . . .

"Hello, Dad . . ."

If Allen heard, he gave no sign.

Jack watched the ubiquitous EKG perform its disconcerting function . . . the IV its rhythmic drip . . .

He bent and kissed his father's dry, slightly stubbly cheek. It felt cold and waxy to the touch. Finally, he reluctantly turned and made his departure, feeling much like a disembodied spirit transporting himself from the nether world . . .

From a pay phone in the foyer, Jack dialed Carolyn's number. There was no answer. He dialed Ben and got an answering device. He dropped the phone on its cradle and turned to go.

But . . . where should he go?

Suddenly Jack felt more alone than ever before . . .

He hesitated. Then reached into his pocket for a coin. As he dialed he realized he was trembling.

"Maria . . . yes, it's Jack. My father's in the hospital. He's very sick . . . may I come over and talk . . .?"

It had taken Maria Ortez ten years to attain the level of independence that she desired. Born in a Juarez barrio, and raised by her widowed mother, some of her earliest memories were of selling trinkets to tourists on the streets. Not for spending money, but to help put beans and rice on the Ortez table.

Maria did not like to remember those days. Nor did she ever want to forget them. She knew from whence she had come. And she was determined never to go back . . .

The secret of how the thin, frightened teenage girl made it across the Border into freedom one moonless night was buried deep in her heart. Maria never spoke of her manumission to anyone. Nor of the infinitely kind lady who rescued her from the streets, who fed her, clothed her, sponsored her and enabled her to achieve U.S. citizenship: one of her lifelong dreams.

Her second most cherished dream was to become a nurse. Not just any nurse. But a nurse who would share love and healing with "the others" — the ones still bound inextricably by the twin chains of ignorance and poverty. Working now as she was, for Drs. Bailey and Drury, this dream was about to manifest.

Nobody could ever know the extent of the appalling struggle it had required for her to make it this far . . .

Maria had found herself in love with Dr. Jack Drury the moment Earl Bailey first brought him into the office. But never, not in her wildest fantasy could she ever imagine Dr. Jack as being even remotely interested in her. How could he be?

The cultural chasm that separated them was far too wide and far too deep . . .

Her heart was pounding when she hung up the telephone. Dr. Jack, coming here? To her apartment? Tonight? To talk about his sick father? But why with me? Why not with Carolyn?

"Madre de Dios," she said aloud.

Maria was not naive. But she was a woman. She knew she was attractive, even pretty. She had heard it often enough . . .

But there was no time to dawdle. He would be here in an hour. Maria was a very clean, fastidious woman and took pride in keeping her tiny apartment sparklingly clean. It was a promise she had made to herself that night she crossed the border.

The only clutter — if it could be called that — were the nursing classes books and papers spread across her coffee table. They took only a moment. She had just returned from class, so she was attractively attired. She took another quick look around. Her house was ready . . .

Now, if only she could still her pounding heart.

Dr. Anne's Journal

She heard footsteps along the walk. The chimes. It must be him. As casually as she could, she opened and let him in. How handsome he looked. But how distraught. His face and eyes bore marks of weariness . . .

"Maria . . . thank you for letting me come. I had to talk with someone. Do you mind if I talk with you? For just a little while . . .?"

"Come in, Dr. Jack. Of course we can talk. Please sit down. May I offer you something? Some chamomile tea perhaps?"

He dropped wearily to a chair. "Yes, Maria. Please. A cup of tea sounds wonderful . . ."

CHAPTER THIRTY

Jack was in a dilemma. With his father hospitalized and out of the picture indefinitely, the power of attorney Allen Drury had drawn up two years prior, which had never been rescinded, made Jack now responsible for his father's practice. Finding himself in professional limbo, Jack contacted Sam Brunson, a semi-retired physician, neighbor and long-time friend of the family.

Sam raked his long, slender fingers through a full head of silvery hair and smiled broadly as he welcomed Jack into his home office. Sam's alert dark eyes twinkled. "Good to see you, Jack, m'boy. What a fine young man you've turned out to be. And fine doctor, I might add . . ."

He leaned back reminiscing. "I remember the time . . ."

He chuckled again and sat up straighter. "But . . . memories are for another day. Tell me, Jack, what can I do for you?"

For a moment Jack, too, was caught up with memories. Sam was ten years older than own his father, and though both doctors were busy with their practices, Sam usually managed to spend regular time with his family each week, something Allen had rarely done.

On more than one occasion Sam had invited Jack to spend the day with him on the golf course, or sailing. Jack never refused.

"We had good times together, Dr. Sam," Jack said. "They meant a great deal to me. And now I have a favor to ask . . ." and then told him the story.

"So you see, Sam," Jack concluded. "I'm in a rather tight spot. Dad's got a good practice, and hundreds of patients depend upon him. Still, at least for the time being, and for who knows how long, you can see that I can't step in and run it . . ."

"Then you're asking me to take over Allen's practice?"

Jack nodded. "Yes . . . for a time at least."

Sam frowned slightly. "You realize, Jack, that I've been on the road for the past year? Lecture tour . . ."

"I hadn't seen you around for months. But I hadn't known about the lecture tour. What's the subject?"

"Glad you asked," Sam said. He handed Jack a small brochure.

NONPRESCRIPTION DRUGS
Proper Use, Misuse And Risks

Dr. Samuel C. Brunson is certified by The American Board of Internal Medicine. He is an honorary clinical professor at UCLA, teaches at Cedars-Sinai and was formerly in private practice in Westwood as an Internist and Endocrinologist.

Dr. Brunson will discuss which over-the-counter drugs (OTCs) may be harmful, ineffective or combine dangerously with other drugs. He will also discuss how to read labels and how to substitute effective, natural, home remedies for OTCs.

> *Dr. Brunson will be appearing
> locally at the following locations and
> dates . . .*

Jack read the brochure quickly and looked up. "So, I guess that means you're not available . . .?" He looked disappointed.

The older physician held up his hand. "What I'm trying to tell you, Jack, is this. It's has been an exciting, productive experience for me. But, just between you and I, I'm tired of getting on and off airplanes for a while. I think I'd enjoy treating patients again . . ."

Then, to Jack's consternation, Sam stood up suddenly and looked at his watch. "Well, what're we waiting for?" he said, placing his arm affectionately around Jack's shoulder.

Jack smiled tentatively, then more broadly than he had in weeks, as the older physician said, "Allen's office should have been opened an hour ago . . ." and began walking him to the door.

"It's breathtaking!" Carolyn said, indicating with her arm the wide sweep of the horizon. "And those clouds, Ben, they're marvelous . . ."

"Yes," Ben said soberly, "I never tire of that view."

They had just returned from a long hike in the mountains and were seated on the deck outside Ben's cabin, with its panoramic view of the Pacific coastline. Carolyn had prepared pita-bread sandwiches, which they were enjoying from lap trays.

Ben wiped his fingers with a napkin. "Carolyn, I'd like to ask a favor of you . . ."

She smiled. "Of course . . . whatever . . ."

Ben wasn't smiling. "It may not be easy . . . but it's very important to me . . ."

Carolyn frowned slightly. "It's okay, Ben. Just . . . ask."

"I don't like to bring up ghosts . . . and I promise this won't be a continuing thing . . ."

She nodded. "You mean, Anne?"

"Yes. I don't know anyone else I can talk to. But, I'd like to talk about . . . well, about her illness. About its genesis. About how . . . well, about the whole cancer bit. Do you mind?"

She thought he looked troubled. Carolyn shook her head slowly. "Not at all, Ben. Let's . . . maybe we can both find answers to some questions. Okay?"

"Thanks . . ."

Ben stood and leaned on the railing, his eyes fixed on a point on the horizon, but Carolyn knew his mind was turning inward . . .

"I don't remember exactly when I first thought Anne was ill," Ben began. "And maybe there wasn't any exact moment. A lot of little things just came together one day. And I knew . . ."

Ben's mind was no longer there on the Malibu hilltop, but was in San Francisco. At Nob Hill. Before Phineas was struck down and died. Even before Magdalene became ill. The four of them had enjoyed a wonderful evening together. After a gourmet dinner they had moved to the library, laughing, talking, listening to Phineas reminisce about some of San Francisco's "early days."

During a lull, Anne said, "I have a question, Grandfather."

"What is it, Anne?" His blue eyes twinkled. "One that you think I can answer?"

Anne laughed and impulsively kissed him on the cheek. "I *know* you can answer it. But nobody else can . . ."

"Oh, a mysterious question?" he teased.

"Something like that . . . it's about your cane. That gold-headed cane that you're never without . . ."

Phineas hefted the object in question. "Yes, child, I've carried this cane for many a mile," he said, stroking the handle. "So . . . what's the question? Where I got it? Who made it?"

She shook her head. "Neither. Since I was a little girl I've thought your cane was, well . . . sort of magical."

Magdalene spoke up. "And as a little girl, you were so very careful not to touch it."

Phineas smiled at the two. How alike they are, he thought: Anne seems like a younger version of her grandmother. "Amazing that you should think about my old cane." He held it up and rotated it slowly, beholding it in different light.

He tucked it between his knees and rested both hands on the head of it, a typical pose, Ben thought.

Phineas looked around at each one, then spoke. "All right, then, I'm ready — *I think* — for the question."

Laughingly Anne said, "Grandfather, I have always thought that the head of your cane was actually a little pistol. I guess you'd call it a derringer. Am I right?"

The old man chuckled. "I don't know how that rumor ever got started . . ."

"Then it's not so?" Anne asked, somewhat crestfallen.

"Yes, child, it is true. My father had it made for him. He carried it on the stage when he rode between here and Sutter's Fort. Protection against bandits. There were a lot of them in '49 and the '50s. Here, I'll show you . . ."

With that, he pressed a concealed latch and the handle came off. In a moment, the gold head was revealed to be a cleverly-designed, double-barrelled derringer. He displayed it fondly, then slid it back and clicked it into place.

"It's never loaded . . ." he explained."It used to be. In the early days. But it hasn't had a cartridge in it for years." "May I see it, Grandfather?" Anne asked and stretched out her hand to receive it . . .

As she reached, Anne suddenly shrieked in pain and quickly slid her right hand to her left armpit. Her face turned suddenly white.

Ben leaped to her side. "Anne . . . what is it?"

In a moment it was over. Color was beginning to return to her face.

"I'm sorry . . ." Anne said. "I . . . I, don't know what happened. Just a sudden stab of pain. I must have twisted my arm the wrong way. I'm all right now . . ."

Nothing more was said that evening. In their bedroom when Ben asked her about it, she brushed it off. "It was nothing . . . just a twinge of some kind. That's all."

Ben moved from the railing and sat beside Carolyn. "I think that was the first inkling I had that Anne was having pain. A number of times after that — when she thought I wasn't watching — I saw her massage that spot under her arm . . ."

"Probably a swollen lymph node," Carolyn said. "Did you notice if the spot was inflamed?"

"Those were my thoughts, too. But Anne was careful not to let me examine it. You see, Anne was really a very private, extremely shy woman . . ."

Carolyn digested that, her eyes idly upon the red-golden sky that presaged a glorious sunset. How could Ben not have noticed an inflamed spot on his wife's body, she wondered.

"I know that sounds strange," Ben was saying, "I mean, for me not to notice things like that. And now I realize I really didn't want to know . . ." Remembering, he sighed. "But she never seemed to be in pain. At least not during those early months of our marriage . . ." He thought about his words, then checked himself.

"Yes, there was something else. I could always tell when she had talked with her father. Collins never communicated with Anne directly. Never called or wrote. But Anne would telephone him once a month or so . . . loyalty, I suppose. Or guilt . . ."

He saw that she had been crying that night when he came into the bedroom, but she hastily retreated to the bathroom, quietly blowing her nose. Moments later when she returned, she was smiling and her face was freshly made up. But there was that dark ring about her eyes. Hollow looking.

"Anne . . ." he began, "what is it?"

"Nothing, really . . . just my time . . . I guess." But she turned her eyes away and wouldn't look at him directly.

He felt anger mounting. "It's your father again, isn't it?"

She nodded and began to cry. He crossed to her and gathered her into his arms, as he had done on so many like occasions.

"He hates me," she said, suddenly in tears. "He hates me. And maybe he's got a right to hate me . . ."

He thrust her away. "What do you mean, Anne? How could your father possibly have any reason to hate you?"

"Because of Mother . . . I . . . I cost him the life of his wife. I took her away from him . . ."

"That's nonsense, Anne. Nonsense. I don't think your father ever loved anyone but himself . . ."

Anne cried all night long. Twice he woke up to the sound of her teeth chattering only to find her shivering and perspiring at the same time . . .

"She was exhausted in the morning," Ben told Carolyn.

Neither of them spoke as they watched the sun's last golden rays fade and Venus begin sparkling in the Western sky. He sought and found her fingers, intertwining his with them.

Carolyn found herself longing to comfort him.

Ben sighed. "About that time Anne began losing weight . . . couldn't do anything about it . . . then she, well . . . she just began to fade away . . ."

"I'm so sorry, Ben . . . so sorry."

Ben nodded.

When he spoke again, it was with a measured tone, with cold, hard anger in his voice. "For a long time I felt guilty about Anne — as though I failed her and allowed her to die . . ."

"No, Ben. No!" She gripped his arm. "No, Ben. It wasn't you. You didn't fail her . . ."

"I *know* that now, Carolyn. But I didn't until I read what she wrote in her journal . . ." He choked with emotion and allowed Carolyn to gently massage his shoulder.

"Until I read what Anne wrote . . . and correlated it with my research. And now I know, Carolyn . . . now I know. Cancer isn't something — some vicious monster — that attacks you from the outside. Cancer comes from the inside . . .

"Cancer is the result of an unhealthy lifestyle — whatever form that may take. Wrong eating, for one. Or habitual gluttony. Lack of exercise. Cancer can be the result of emotional trauma — anger, rage, unforgiveness, unrelieved stress . . .

"In fact, I believe that unrelieved conflict of any kind can cause cancer. Some researchers even think cancer is connected to parental conflict or disapproval, perceived even in the womb.

"And God knows," Ben went on slowly, "Anne felt that disapproval all her life . . ."

He looked at her. "Carolyn, you're a nurse. And you already know some of these things. But I've got to say them. To get the words out of my mind. Okay?"

"Of course," she whispered.

"I believe that even fear can result in cancer. Loneliness and rejection cause cancer. Feelings of unworth can eventually cause cancer . . .

"Carolyn, all of her life, Anne was plagued with those negative emotions. Those damned detrimental, destructive emotions! Then I came into her life and she felt — she wrote it in her journal — she felt like my love would compensate and enable her body to rebuild her and to make her whole. And it would have . . . it *could have*, except for one thing . . ."

"What was that?" Carolyn whispered. "What was that?"

"Even then she was emotionally incapable of controlling her own life. Her own destiny . . ."

"But, I don't understand?" Carolyn said.

"It seems so obvious now. But I didn't catch onto it in time. Collins controlled Anne. He called every shot. Directed her every move. And she continued to let him do it. He even got Drury to hire her. No matter what she did, no matter where she was, Collins kept a tight rein on Anne. He wouldn't let her go. He destroyed her by default . . .

"But that wasn't all he did . . ." Ben pounded the redwood rail with his fists, emphasizing each word. "Collins forbade Anne from using alternative therapy!"

Ben dropped to his knees on the deck.

Without a word, Carolyn knelt beside him. Their tears mixed and ran together and dripped on the sun-dried wood, leaving stains that would remain for a long time.

329

CHAPTER THIRTY-ONE

Earl Bailey had his hands full. With Jack Drury out of the office, his patient load suddenly doubled. A few of Jack's patients he could handle, but many required the services of a medical doctor. Of major concern to Bailey was the problem concerning the handful of desperately ill patients who depended entirely upon Drury. They suddenly found themselves cast adrift with nowhere to go.

"You've got to help me do something," Bailey told Jack over the telephone. "I'm drowning . . . patients are suffering . . ."

"Earl, my hands have been tied by the courts. I don't know what I can do."

"At least come to the office and let's talk about it. There must be some kind of a solution to our dilemma . . ."

Jack thought about that. "Okay, Earl, I'll come. But it'll have to be after hours, when there are no patients around. Maybe we can come up with something . . ."

Maria was still in the front office when he arrived. She smiled shyly. "We miss you around here, Doctor Jack . . ."

He grinned ruefully. "No more than I miss being here, Maria. Is Doc still around?"

She shrugged toward the hallway. "Back in his office. Trying to get caught up with his paper work

. . ." She indicated her desk that was piled high. "So am I."

She sighed. "It just keeps piling up . . ." Her eyes filled with tears. "And the sick people keep coming . . . We need so very much for you to be here . . . and I . . ."

Maria didn't finish the sentence. Nor did she have to. Jack knew what she meant. Neither of them could forget that evening together. Nor did they want to . . .

Jack patted her shoulder. "I know, Maria. I know . . . I hope something will soon work out. Light a candle for me . . . for all of us, okay?"

Maria nodded and watched him stride down the familiar hallway to Bailey's tiny office. Just seeing him, and hearing his voice lifted her spirits. Would he come again?

Bailey looked exhausted. He started to rise, but Jack waved him down. "Don't get up, Earl. I think I know how you feel . . ."

"It's only been two weeks, Jack . . . seems like a year."

Jack leaned back. "Any ideas?"

"Not a single one. I've been combing my tired brain. So far I've come up with a big fat zero. How about you?" He grinned hopefully.

"Maybe. Maybe not." He opened his brief case and pulled out a lined yellow pad. He glanced briefly at his notes, then looked up. "Truth is, I *do* have some ideas that I'd like to toss around."

"I'm open to about anything short of witchcraft . . ."

Jack chuckled mirthlessly. "Depends who hears what I've got to say . . . some would think it is witchcraft . . ."

"Oh?" Bailey pulled himself to an upright position. "Bad as that? Or, as good?"

"Who knows . . ." Jack answered slowly, while he doodled figure eights on the top of his pad. "Well, anyway, Earl, I've been thinking, this boondoggle just *might be* the best thing that ever happened to you . . . to us . . ."

Bailey sucked in his breath. "You're not kidding, are you?"

"No, Earl, I'm not." He tapped his pencil on the pad. "You see, I've got a list here of some other holistic practitioners we might consider . . ."

"I don't get you. Like what?" Bailey asked.

"I'm saying, why don't we build this clinic into a multi-disciplinary medical center?"

Bailey opened his mouth to speak, but Jack stopped him.

"Now, hold on, before you answer, hear me out. If, besides you and I, that is, a chiropractor and a medical physician, we'd get us a homeopathic physician, and a naturopath . . ."

"And an acupuncturist and a psychologist . . ." Bailey interjected, a wide grin spreading across his weary face. "We could truly cover all the bases, all the modalities . . ."

"Exactly," Jack said, "all of methods of healing have a great deal to offer. So, why not pull them all together. Each one an equal partner on the same basis that you and I work on . . ."

"That's a great idea!" Bailey said, then, more somberly. "Yeah, but what about you?"

"I've thought about that, too. And I think I've even got that figured out . . ." He doodled some more before he spoke. "I've done some talking with a couple of the doctors in the Tijuana clinics. Both American and Mexican. And I think they might find a place for me to practice with them . . ."

With gradual comprehension, Bailey's eyes lit up again. "I think I get the picture," he said. "We could have the best of both worlds. We — the other doctors and I — could treat most patients right here. And the ones we couldn't treat within the parameters of existing medical restrictions . . . those we would send to you. Is that it?"

"You get the picture . . ."

Bailey's face clouded. "But, who knows when you'd be able to come back here to practice?"

"Based on the information I've gotten from several practitioners who have been treated like me," Jack said slowly, "it could be a long-drawn out affair, months or even years. And even then, after all that time and money, the authorities might *still* prevent me from practicing medicine in the United States."

"So, what are you thinking?" Bailey asked.

"Maybe I won't even try to buck the system myself. Maybe it wouldn't be worth it in the long run. Maybe I'll just practice medicine in Mexico and let it go at that . . ."

He shrugged. "But then again, if I don't fight, I'll be letting down all the sick people who are depending upon me . . . the ones with no options. I just don't know . . ."

Jack slid his papers back into his attache case. "Right now I've got a little time to work on this idea . . . so, I thought I'd make some phone calls, talk to a few people. Okay?"

Bailey grinned his old familiar grin. "Let's go for it!"

On the way out, Jack bent and whispered in Maria's ear. She nodded her answer and turned quickly back to her work lest he see the bright color rising in her olive cheeks. Later, Bailey heard her singing softly . . .

Nob Hill wasn't the same without Phineas and Magdalene. Or Anne. But Ben loved the Nob, even apart from the lovely people in his life who had made it home for him. Until they had purchased the Malibu cabin, the Nob had been Anne's most favorite place in all the world. She had loved to stand at the

living room window and watch the fog roll across the
Bay . . .

He had never seen the Bay from this
perspective before, and she had introduced him to the
wonder of it all when they spent their first Holiday
together at the Nob. Even then, had he been astute
enough, Ben might have detected an early harbinger
of what was to come . . .

"This is my most *favoritest* place," she said.

"Nob Hill?"

She shook her head. "Nob Hill, yes. But,
actually, right here. At this window . . ."

"I don't understand?"

"It's the fog, Ben. The fog. It rolls over
everything. Takes over everything. Nothing can
prevent it. Nothing. Not life . . . not even death . . ."

For a moment he imagined he heard a morose
quality in her voice he'd never heard before. Then he
looked at her, and to his astonishment, two large
tears coursed down her cheeks . . .

"Why, Anne . . . my dear? Is something . . .?"

She shook her head. "Nothing is wrong, Ben.
It's the fog. It always does this to me . . . it's like,
well, it's like a huge *something*, something without a
name . . . it just rolls over the Bay, and it's gone.
Death does that, Ben, it just rolls over a person . . .
and they are gone . . ."

He pondered that conversation for days.

Standing now in that same spot with Carolyn,
beholding the same awe inspiring phenomenon, Ben
pondered that conversation with Anne. Even then, he
thought, she must have known, or at least had an
inkling of what was to be . . .

Neither Ben nor Carolyn spoke as San
Francisco Bay displayed its remarkable tableau . . .

One moment the sky was clear and blue, with
only scattered fleecy clouds scudding about, pierced
on the north by the Golden Gate's towering pylons.
To the east Alcatraz squatted, grey, lonely and

forbidding. Rumor had it, Ben remembered, that only two desperate prisoners had ever swum to freedom from the Rock. Or had they been devoured by sharks? No one knew.

To the right of Alcatraz lay Treasure Island and the Oakland Bay Bridge . . . the entire Bay dotted with whitecaps and multi-colored sails . . .

Moments later, the invincible fog rolled through the Golden Gate, enveloping pylons and towers, Angel Island, Alcatraz and all the rest, as legions of horns, bells and whistles reverberated their cacophonous warnings . . .

Relentless tendrils of the almighty fog crept up the hill, resisted only by the window behind which Ben and Carolyn stood.

Released from the Bay's hypnotic demonstration of invincible power, Carolyn sighed. "It's wonderful. Magnificent . . ."

"Yes," Ben replied nostalgically. "It's always like that."

"Oh, Ben, this is a marvelous home . . . awesome, really."

Ben nodded.

He had brought Carolyn here for a reason . . .

Practically all of the research was completed, with only a few loose ends to tie up. "It will take me months to write it," he told Carolyn one evening, ". . . and when I write, I do little of anything else. I write, sleep a little, eat some, then write some more. It's a cycle . . ."

"Vicious cycle?" she teased.

"It tends to get pretty vicious. So . . ." he said, "there's something I want to do before I begin."

"What's that?" Carolyn asked, puzzled by his solemnity.

"I want to put some ghosts to bed."

"More ghosts?" she smiled.

He wasn't smiling. "Yes, more ghosts . . . in San Francisco. And I'd like for you to come with me. Will you?"

Her eyes didn't waver. "Yes, Ben, if that's what you want me to do. Yes, I'll go . . ."

Now they were here and he didn't know quite where to begin.

CHAPTER THIRTY-TWO

Those first two days had been the hardest. Even though they gave him all the water and vegetable juice he wanted — gallons, it seemed — they had withheld solid food. "That's to prepare you for the diagnostic tests," the nurse told him. Now, after several weeks in the clinic, Ted was a different person.

"I haven't felt this good in years," he told Toni. "You haven't looked this good either . . ."

Shaffer remembered that long drive to Tijuana as being the most painful experience of his life. No matter how he tried to brace himself in the back seat of Jack's suburban sedan, he was unable to fully protect himself against the constant jolting of the stop and go traffic. And, miles before they reached their destination, Ted was in agony.

"Doctor, I just can't take it any longer," he moaned. "You've just got to stop . . ."

Jack pulled off at the first offramp, and catheterized Ted to relieve the pressure. For most of the rest of the way he was able to sleep, while Jack and Toni sat in the front and talked.

"I'm very grateful . . ." Toni said.

Jack grinned as he expertly tooled the vehicle in the now thinning traffic. "Think nothing of it . . ."

"But, we're both grateful, Doctor."

To change the subject, Jack asked, "How long have you been aware of your husband's difficulty?"

"About two years, I think. At first he had difficulties only at night . . . he had to get up three or four times to go to the bathroom. But neither one of us thought much about it . . ."

"Did he have much pain then?" Jack asked.

"No. Just discomfort. It was several months before he had what he actually called pain . . ."

"Any blood in the urine?"

She shook her head. "I don't know. He didn't tell me. And, I guess I was afraid to ask. Afraid what he might tell me . . ."

Toni was not a pretty woman, but she had taken good care of herself and wore her years well. She was obviously devoted to her husband, and he to her.

"Do you think Ted has a good chance . . . of . . .?" She was unable to complete the sentence.

Jack smiled at her. "He showed me copies of the tests that Dr. Spicer took. And, to be perfectly honest . . ."

She interrupted. "We do want that. Perfect honesty. Okay?"

"Of course. To be perfectly honest, Ted is in a serious condition. He waited far too long . . . the prostate is enlarged and has practically shut off the neck of the bladder . . ."

"What can be done?" she asked timorously. "Will he still have to have surgery?"

Jack shrugged. "Toni, I don't personally know. But, I can assure you that everything will be done to avoid it . . ."

He pointed to a freeway sign. "We're almost to Carlsbad. Do you want to stop and eat?"

Toni looked back at Ted, who was still sleeping. She shook her head. "No. Not unless you are hungry. I'd like to get him to the clinic before he wakes up . . ."

"Good. We have enough fuel to make it all the way . . ."

Apparently something was bothering Toni. She started to talk several times, then said nothing. Finally, Jack said, "Toni, if you have any questions . . . any at all . . . please ask them. I think it might relieve your mind . . ."

She took a deep breath. "Yes, Doctor, I would like to ask you something . . . the . . . treatment . . . is it going to be painful? I mean, really painful?"

He shook his head. "No. Other than drawing blood for tests, and needle punctures for IVs — multivitamins, enzymes and the like — I don't think he'll be uncomfortable at all . . ."

"Uh, Doctor . . ."

"Yes?" Jack saw that she was blushing.

"Just one more question. It's sort of personal . . . if you don't mind . . .?"

"Anything. Go ahead."

"Doctor, will it be alright again . . . I mean for the two of us? I mean, will he . . . will Ted . . .?"

His eyes were twinkling. "Toni, I believe it's going to be alright . . . for both of you. In every way . . ."

She leaned back and relaxed against the seat cushion. "Thanks, Doctor . . . thanks for understanding."

They were nearing San Diego now and traffic was heavier. Jack was very intent upon his driving for a few minutes. "There is something, though, that might be difficult . . ."

Toni sat up straighter. "What's that?"

"His eating situation. I judge from what Ted told me, that he used to eat a lot of meat . . . desserts . . . drink a lot of coffee. Sort of the standard American diet. Is that right?"

"Yes. I'd rather have more fresh things. You know, salads, fresh fruit, things like that. But Ted always told me, 'You eat that rabbit food if you want . . . but I'm a meat and potatoes man.' So," she gestured helplessly, "I fed him what he wanted."

She sighed and spoke wistfully. "But, he hasn't eaten much of anything these past months . . . no appetite . . . and he's lost so much weight . . ."

"I think that will change," Jack said brightly. "I think he'll begin eating again. But his diet will have to change. You know that. And it'll no longer be a matter of what he might have wanted to eat. If his body is going to heal itself, he'll have to give it the building materials his body needs . . ."

She picked up on that. "Do you really think Ted's body is going to heal itself?"

"Yes, Toni. Yes, I do." He moved his right hand from the wheel and gripped hers. "I believe Ted's going to get well. He's got a strong will. And a devoted, determined wife . . ."

He smiled at her. "All that's in Ted's favor. Yes, I believe he'll make it . . ."

Ted and Toni Shaffer were sitting together in the sun, on the veranda outside the clinic. "I don't have any more pain," Ted was saying. "I've got an appetite for the first time in . . . how long has it been? Months? Years?"

Toni nodded happily. "It's been a long time, Ted. There's something else about you now . . . you seem so . . . happy. And that makes me happy, too. I think it's wonderful. Because these past six or eight months it hasn't been that way. You've seemed so, I don't know, down . . . discouraged . . ."

He chuckled. "It's because I was discouraged. Life wasn't fun anymore." He bent over and kissed her. "You were always there for me . . . but I wasn't there for you. I'm sorry . . ."

"But," he said with a big grin, "all that's changed now. For the better . . . I just talked to the doctor . . ."

"Oh . . . What did he say?" The barest trace of a worry wrinkle showed between Toni's eyes.

"Well, for one, he told me all my tests are normal. Not a trace of cancer in my blood . . . he said I can go home in a week. He told me I've got to keep on eating — and taking the supplements — like I've been doing down here."

He made a face. "But, I can do that. It's worth all of it to be alive, really alive again . . ."

Toni clapped her hands like a schoolgirl. "Oh, Ted . . . I'm so happy!"

Ted grinned impishly. "He told me something else . . ."

"What was that?"

"The doctor told me . . . that I could be a married man again . . ."

Despite herself, Toni felt the color rise to her cheeks.

"Carolyn," Ben spoke softly, "I've always said that when you don't know where to begin . . . that the best way is to begin at the beginning."

"I know," she smiled, "you have told me that."

He nodded absently. "Anyway, there are some things that I must do . . . some thinking I've got to sort out, that could only be done here, in San Francisco . . ."

"And ghosts . . .?"

"Yes, and ghosts to put to rest." He regarded her intently. "And I needed to talk some of them out with you . . ."

"Well, here we are. Let's go."

Like turning back pages in a book, Ben leapfrogged the years to when he was in high school. Sports he loved, but the library was his friend. Others memorized baseball scores; Ben mastered the Dewey decimal system and the card catalog. Physiology and anatomy drew him like twin magnets. Along with all that had to do with either, or both.

"You will become a doctor," the librarian once prophesied.

He doggedly shook his head. "No. I'm going to be a writer."

She looked puzzled. "But the books you read . . .?"

"That's what I'm going to write about . . ."

His father despaired. His mother glowed. His friends were mostly "jocks." They called him "Doc." But, as it turned out, he hadn't written about the body, or health, or medicine. Somewhere along he'd gotten sidetracked and had begun writing short stories — mystery short stories. They began selling. He moved to books. They sold . . . and then he was slotted . . .

"So, actually," he was telling Carolyn, "it wasn't until Anne became ill that I thought very much about my earlier love. And now . . ." he shrugged, "that's all I want to write about. I seem almost to be driven . . ."

"Driven?" Carolyn asked. "Driven to do what?"

"Well, it started out with Anne's death. I felt compelled to try and find out the truth about her death . . . well, actually, the truth about why she refused the treatment she must have known could have saved her life. That's where it started . . ."

"And now?"

"That's just it . . . now that I'm learning some answers to my questions . . . well, then I keep asking more questions . . ."

Restlessly, Ben jumped and paced back and forth before the bay window, now grey with fog. "It seems that I'm driven to know even more. I now believe that Anne died of cancer because she was unable to free herself from her emotional quagmire of anger, fear and guilt. And because of that, she simply could not choose the therapy that was best for her . . .

"Dr. Deepak Chopra articulated that concept very well in his book, *Quantum Healing*.[59] He said, 'cure of cancer . . . depends on a special quality of mind, some deep will to live, a heroically positive outlook. . . . The reason why not everyone manages to take the healing process as far as it can go is that we differ drastically in our ability to mobilize it.'"

Ben paused, then went on slowly. "Anne was a special woman. But she still was unable to overcome the detrimental effects of her father's hold on her. And thus could not adequately mobilize the totality of her body's healing processes . . ."

He dropped his head as though to clarify his mind. "But my quest hasn't stopped by quantifying the forces that destroyed her. I had to learn how she developed cancer in the first place. I don't believe it was genetically caused. Nor even that it was a nutritional problem . . . especially in the beginning."

Carolyn had risen and was pacing with him, step for step. "Okay, if it was neither genetic nor nutritional in her case, then what was the cause?"

"I believe," Ben said, "that Anne's cancer began when she was a little girl. I have thought that for a long time. And it had something to do with the way life impacted her immune system. That's becoming very clear to me now . . . the distillation of everything I have read and heard about the immune system . . .

"I believe the immune system is much more than a bunch of organs working in concert. I believe the immune system is an accurate reflection, a mirror image of the life within, and that it responds to everything in one's life: to its joys and anguish, to its exuberance and boredom, laughter and tears, its excitement and depression, its problems and prospects . . .

"In fact, Carolyn," Ben said, "I believe that there is scarcely anything that enters or affects the mind that does not in some way affect the intricate workings of the body . . ."

Ben stopped pacing and stared unseeingly into the fog bank, through which a few brave lights were

valiantly attempting to illumine the way for foot and
auto traffic. Carolyn nodded, but did not speak.

"As a little girl," Ben went on, "Anne had no
control over her life. None whatever. She had no
choice in what she would wear, or eat, or where she
would go to school. She was raised by strangers. Her
own father withheld his love. He never touched her.
She thought it was because she had caused her
mother's death and that he hated her for that . . .

"So, early on, desperately striving to earn her
father's affection, and continuously failing to do the
single thing she wanted to do, her body got the
message, and began to die. So, you see, I am
beginning to agree with a growing number of
physicians and scientists such as Dr. Bernie Siegel
. . ."

"The famous cancer surgeon?"

"Yes. In one of his books he wrote an entire
chapter on the subject.[60] Woody Allen summed up the
idea well with one of his famous lines, when he said,
'I can't express anger. I internalize it and grow a
tumor instead.'

"But Bernie Siegel expressed what, is to me,
the saddest thing I know — especially since it
describes the tragedy of Anne so clearly and
succinctly . . ."

He stopped speaking and Carolyn saw tears
running down his cheeks. She stepped close to him
and her arm around his waist. "What did he say?"
she asked gently.

Ben sighed. "Bernie states a universal truth —
that the goal of the human mind is peace . . . And
with all my heart, I believe he is right. The thing
that is so sad is not until she met me did Anne ever
experience even a modicum of the peace she
desperately sought . . .

"Achieving that goal of peace, Siegel said, will
give the body the message that it is supposed to
live.[61] However, he didn't explicitly state the flip side

of that statement, which is just as true . . . If one's mind never finds peace, it gives the body just the opposite message . . .

"So, you see, Carolyn . . ." Ben said, shaking his head sadly, "for over thirty years, Anne's mind sent that negative message to her body. And by the time she and I found each other her body had already — long before, in fact — begun to act upon that message . . ."

"But, weren't you and Anne happy?" Carolyn asked.

"Happy, yes. But for Anne, peaceful, no. Her father never let go . . . emotionally he never relinquished his grip upon her mind. He never allowed her to experience peace . . . and so the message Anne's mind sent her body never changed . . ."

Ben resumed pacing again, this time with Carolyn's fingers entwined with his own. They paced for several minutes in silence — twenty paces and turn, twenty paces and turn.

"As you might know," he finally said, his words spoken in cadence with his pacing, "I've been reading everything I could find on cancer. Cancer and it's healing, or cure, whichever you want to call it . . .

"I've studied all kinds of therapies, modalities, protocols, you name it. Even faith healing and what some doctors call spontaneous remission. Some even call it spontaneous cure . . . And I've learned a lot . . ."

He gave her a quick sidelong glance and caught his breath. He had never studied her profile before. It was classically beautiful. Her lips were slightly parted, and her long lashes were silhouetted against the window. The damp atmosphere had formed little ringlets of her hair. Intent upon his words, she was unaware of his *coup d'oeil* . . .

As he picked up where he left off, he wondered if she could hear the rapid drum beat of his heart. "I have always believed in the close connection between the mind and the body. And the strong influence one's thoughts and attitudes exercise over one's health . . ."

He paused and Carolyn responded quickly. "Oh, yes . . . I agree. I believe one's will is all important."

He nodded. "Yes, but there must be freedom to develop that will. And the will to live, to defeat all obstacles, to overcome any foe, must be developed . . . and allowed to grow . . . and when it does not have that freedom, I believe the deep inner spirit atrophies . . . a terrible, terrible condition . . ."

There came a knock at the library door and Mrs. Oberley, the Elias' long-time housekeeper, peeked in. "Excuse me, Ben, but would you and the lady like some dinner?"

"Would you care to eat?" Ben asked.

Carolyn laughingly placed both hands across her abdomen. "Yes . . . I'm starved . . ."

"Would you mind serving us in here?" he asked.

"Not a'tall. About fifteen minutes?"

"Carolyn," Ben said, after they had eaten and were warming themselves before the snapping-crackling fire, "I'm telling you all this for several reasons. One, because I want to remove all the ghosts from my life. I had to do that here in San Francisco. That's where most of them were.

"Two, I needed a sounding board for many of the thoughts that have been bombarding my brain for so long . . . I think you understand those thoughts. You're a medical person . . . and you're a woman . . ."

Chapter Thirty-Two

He turned and faced her directly. "The third reason, I believe, is the most important of all . . ." He paused and fixed her with a steady look.

Carolyn held his level gaze with external cool composure, but inside she was anything but calm. "And just what is your third reason?" she asked.

He drew a deep breath, held it, and exhaled it slowly. He treated her to his warm gentle smile. "I think you already know the answer to *that* question. Don't you?"

She nodded. "Yes, Ben, I think I do . . ."

CHAPTER THIRTY-THREE

"I challenge you to give me the name of *anybody* who's been cured of cancer," the young man said angrily. "Cancer is genetic. It runs in families. I should know. My mother, my father and my sister all died of cancer. My grandfather died of cancer. And, I have every right to expect that I'll die of cancer . . .

"Furthermore," he sneered, "the *natural means* you're talking about are phony. Everything's phony they use on cancer. Might as well let cancer run its course. Once you get it you're going to die anyway. Nothing's going to change that!"

Ben flinched at the intensity of the challenge. Until less than an hour ago he had never heard the name, Oscar Bjork. He and Ross Hannibal were leaving the cable TV station where the two of them had granted an interview concerning Ben's forthcoming book when Bjork accosted them.

The security guard tried to restrain the heckler, but Ben waved him away. "We'll be happy to talk to this man," he said. Turning to Ross, he asked, "May we go to your office?"

Thirty minutes later, seated in the comfortable conference room at Cutting Edge Publications, Ben allowed Bjork to run down before he spoke.

"Before I try to answer your questions," Ben began, "let's get two or three things clear. First, I am not a doctor. I'm a writer, an investigative writer. Second, concerning the genetic nature of cancer . . .

that's up for grabs. Very controversial and unproven. Then, third, when we're finished talking, if you want them, I can give you the names of a number of people who have been healed of cancer . . ."

Bjork interrupted, "Nobody's been cured of . . ."

"Hold it!" Ben said. "Let me finish. And, let me remind you that you've never heard me use the word cure . . ."

"You said *healed*. It means the same thing," Bjork countered. "Just semantics . . ."

Ben shook his head. "Let me explain again. To me, and to most people, the word *cured* conjures up the picture of a drug or other substance, that will remove the cancer symptoms . . ."

"You're evading the point . . ." Bjork began.

"Hold on," Ross commanded. "Mr. Rush allowed you to speak your piece. Now you either listen to him or leave . . ."

Bjork angrily settled himself down in his chair.

"If that's what you or anyone means by a *cure* for cancer," Ben went on, "then there is no cure for cancer. Which means it can't be cured.

"However . . . if the *causes* of cancer are removed, then there is every reason to believe the condition can be reversed. Or eliminated. In that case, I would say that the patient had been healed of cancer."

"Or the cancer's in remission!" Bjork burst out.

Ben shrugged. "What's the difference? If the remission lasts for ten years, twenty years, or fifty years, at what point would you say the cancer had been healed? Or would you?"

"And I suppose you've got some names of such people?"

"Yes, I do. Along with their addresses and telephone numbers?"

"And I can contact them?"

Ben smiled pleasantly. "Of course. Let me just share one example of what I'm talking about. Burgess

Parks is a remarkable older gentleman who managed
to heal himself of cancer . . ."

At the age of 71, Burgess Parks was diagnosed
with colon cancer, and during the next few months
underwent four major surgeries in an effort to save
his life. In the process, the surgeon removed two
malignant tumors, one the size of an orange, and 12
inches of his colon.

"According to Burgess' wife, Mary June," Ben
said, "that was when the doctors sent him home to
die. But Burgess Parks didn't die. And, as of this
moment — some 13 years later, Burgess is 84 years
old and *very much alive* . . .

"Furthermore," Ben added, "for the majority of
those years, the Parks have driven their motor home
from coast to coast each year telling hundreds of
thousands of people that it's possible to be healed of
cancer."

"How did he heal himself?" Ross asked.

"Mary June Parks describes the whole process
in her four books,"[62] Ben said, "but basically Burgess
regained his health and the two of them remain
healthy by instituting a radical change of lifestyle,
including their diet.

"And in a recent, personal letter, Mary June
Parks said, 'In addition to what we removed from
Burgess' diet, we added lots of raw vegetable juices
and raw foods, home-made, whole-grain breads and
cereals. All this, including a strong program of
supplements, enabled Burgess to regain his strength
almost immediately . . .'"

"And that's it?" Bjork asked.

"No. Not at all. The healing process took time.
The man's strength, according to his wife, came back
almost immediately. But it was months before
Burgess became a healthy man again. But, to answer
your question more fully, the Parks keep their bodies
supplied with plenty of fresh oxygen and they
exercise properly.

"'Besides that,' Mary June says, 'we maintain a positive mental attitude and a true spirit of forgiveness. We manifest a strong desire to live, and we allow God's healing energies to flow . . .'"[63]

Ben handed Bjork the promised list. "That's about it. Now you can check all this out for yourself . . ."[64]

It was quickly evident to Carolyn that she and Dr. Brunson were philosophically on the same wave length regarding health and healing. When their last patient left that first day, Brunson invited Carolyn into his office. He pulled off his coat, laced his fingers behind his head and leaned back in his chair.

"Mind if I drop the Miss, and just call you Carolyn?" Brunson asked with the characteristic twinkle in his eyes. "After all, I am old enough to be your father . . ."

She laughed comfortably. "Please do. I'd like that."

"And . . ." he continued, "if you'd like to call me Dr. Sam, or just plain Sam . . . I'll answer to either one . . ."

He regarded her thoughtfully. "Jack told me a lot about you, Carolyn. I liked what he said. And I like what I've seen today. And, since it looks like I might be here for some time, probably several months at least, we should get acquainted . . ."

Brunson leaned forward with his elbows on the desk. "So, why don't we just talk a bit. Okay?"

Carolyn smiled affably. "Mind if I kick off my shoes?"

His laughter was her answer.

"I believe in letting the patient tell me what his or her problems are, and then listening while they talk," Brunson said. "After all, the patient knows better than I do where he or she hurts. In the long run, I think I've learned more from my patients than they have learned from me . . ."

He picked up a handful of drug samples from the desk and eyed them curiously. "Drugs . . . if used properly and not to excess, can be helpful. Or, they can become a crutch and a curse. Would you agree?"

"Very much so, Dr. Brunson . . . I mean, Dr. Sam . . ."

Brunson stood up and stretched. "I've been doctoring for a good many years . . . and I've learned a lot."

He grinned boyishly. "Still got a lot to learn. But I've learned that many patients have the attitude, 'Doctor, I don't want to change the way I live. Just give me a shot. Or something. Just fix me up and let me live my life the way I've been doing it.'"

He loosened his tie and removed it. "Carolyn, those patients don't come back to me very often . . . do you know why?"

She smiled. "I think I can guess."

"What would you guess?"

"I think you'd tell them they've got to take responsibility for their own health. I think you'd tell them that drugs and medicine can't heal bodies that have been damaged by bad living habits. And that only right living, coupled with right attitudes can heal."

"You've got it. I tell them that if they'll work with me, that between us, we'll have a good chance of helping them to get well. But if they're not willing to help me to help them . . . well, then, they'd just better seek another opinion . . ."

Brunson pulled out a patient's chart and gave it a cursory glance. "These things are important. Really important." He looked up. "Do you feel, comfortable taking a patient's history, or what I call a health biography?"

"Well, yes . . ." she said, "at least the basics . . ."

Dr. Anne's Journal

"Good," he said "let's work as a team. If you'll obtain a solid health biography from patients, I can do my job better."

"Dr. Sam . . ." Carolyn began, "a health biography could cover a lot of territory. Just how much of it do you want me to cover?"

Brunson grinned. "Good question." He handed her a folder. "Here, this will help you. As you can see, I've developed a rather comprehensive health biography form . . . I don't expect you to cover all of it with the patients, but it will give you some idea of what I need to take it from there . . ."

As Carolyn was opening the folder, Dr. Sam said, "Of course, as you can see, it begins with the usual questions . . . the immediate complaints . . . the ones that brought the patient to our office . . .

"But, that's just for starters. Going beyond that, I'd like know how happy the patient is. Something about his or her home life . . . work life . . . social life . . ."

"I get the idea," Carolyn said. "What you're really trying to determine is the *causes* that brought on the symptoms . . ."

"That's it exactly. Then we can to do what I call 'fine tuning,' and begin rectifying the problem. Then we won't simply be treating the symptoms . . ."

Carolyn broke in, "At that point you will be treating the causes. Right?"

"You've got it, Carolyn. And though the patient may not know it at the time, that's exactly what he or she needs . . . But when we reach that point in our therapy, everybody is a winner — especially the patients."

Ross Hannibal skillfully cut the engine and eased the *Blue Pencil* into its Marina Del Rey slip. The instant the bow touched the dock, Ben leaped ashore and secured the bow and stern lines to the cleats, then climbed back aboard and helped Ross secure and store the sails.

"Ben, you're becoming a regular salt," Ross observed.

"Thanks . . . I've got an excellent skipper. And, thanks, Ross, it's been a wonderfully relaxing weekend . . ."

By mid-Friday afternoon, after a long week at his computer, Ben had found himself infected with such a rare, but virulent case of "writer's block," that the words he was generating were no longer flowing as they ought.

He dialed Carolyn, "How about a weekend in San Francisco?"

"Ben, I'd love to. But Dr. Sam and I've got our hands full for all day tomorrow. I'm so sorry . . ."

He groaned. "I've got to get away from this computer for a few days . . ."

"Why don't you call Ross Hannibal?" she suggested, knowing that the two of them loved to sail.

"Great idea. I'll do that. But, Carolyn . . ." he paused.

"Yes, Ben . . . what is it?"

"Please make arrangements for next weekend. Let's fly up to on Friday evening . . . and come back Monday morning. Okay? I've got something very important to discuss with you . . ."

Carolyn shivered with anticipation. "I'll talk to Dr. Sam right now. Let's count on it . . ."

Ben dialed Ross's office. He'd barely said hello when Ross said, "My bag's packed for the weekend, Ben. And I'm looking for my crew. Are you available?"

"Am I ever! I'll meet you at the marina within the hour."

After they had carefully maneuvered their way through the Friday evening marina traffic, and had passed the breakwater, Ross said, "Ben, take the

wheel . . . I'm going to prepare us a whopping good
meal fit for any captain and his first mate!"

The *Blue Pencil* was a smart craft and
responded beautifully to the helm. The snapping of
her taut sails was music to Ben's ears. It felt good
again to taste the salt spray on his lips and to brace
himself against the pitch and roll of the open sea.

Even before Ross stuck his head through the
hatch and shouted, "Chow down," Ben was sensing
his accumulated stresses beginning to dissipate.

"The synopsis of your book is top notch," Ross
told Ben later as they were beating their way due
westward into the setting sun.

"Thanks . . ."

"And I presume the writing's going well?"

"Yes . . . and no . . . you know how that goes
. . ."

Ross nodded and tossed a bread crust to a sea
gull and chuckled as it swooped to catch it before it
struck the water.

"But, I've got a question . . "

"Oh, what's that?" Ross asked.

"Nothing much to do with the book . . . and
maybe you don't want to tackle it . . ."

"And why not?"Ross asked. "Too tough for me?"

His eye on the compass, Ben moved the wheel
a spoke to keep on course. "Not that. It's a theological
question. One that Anne asked in her journal . . ."

"What's the question?"

"Well, before Anne's grandmother died," Ben
began slowly, feeling his way, "both her grandparents
were praying that God would deliver the woman and
let her live. But she died . . .

"And then, when Anne became ill, she was
praying that God would deliver her . . ."

"And *she* died," Ross finished softly.

Ben nodded.

"So you want me to tell you why God didn't
answer their prayers? Is that it?"

Ben nodded again. A sudden gust struck the full sails and the *Blue Pencil* heeled, taking water over the lee rail. Ben gripped the wheel with both hands to hold her steady.

Ross spoke above the rising wind. "Ben, what would have happened if you'd released control of the helm just then?"

Ben looked puzzled. "We'd have probably swamped. And unless somebody rescued us, we might have drowned. Why?"

"Even if you had prayed for God to take control of the helm when you released it . . .?"

Comprehension dawned. "That's it, Ross. That's it! It was so simple and plain that I didn't see it . . ."

"Tell me about it."

"I was in charge of the helm, Ross. I was responsible for the steering and safety of the boat . . ."

Keeping a steady hand on the helm, he took a quick look at Ross. "Right so far?"

"Right on, Ben."

"That means, that if I had let go of the helm — either purposely or negligently, or in ignorance, even if I had prayed and asked God to take over the steering — it would have been my fault, and mine alone, if the boat got into trouble. Right?"

"That's right, Ben. God tells us repeatedly that He will be with us. But nowhere in the Bible does God tell us that He will take responsibility for something that we could do, or could have done, but didn't."

Ben sighed grimly. "I understand. Anne had researched other modalities for treating her cancer. But, because of fear of her father, or for whatever other reasons, she failed to act upon the knowledge she had . . ."

Dr. Anne's Journal

"Yes," Ross said gently, "and like it or not, Ben, that made her — not God, not you — responsible for her choices . . ."

Recent rain had washed San Francisco clean and bright as a new penny and receding thunder clouds were retreating seaward as the American Airlines jet dropped over the Bay and touched down. Ben retrieved Carolyn's carry-on luggage from the overhead rack and they quickly disembarked.

Ben had phoned ahead and their car and driver awaited them at the curb. "Welcome back to San Francisco, Ben," the chauffeur said warmly.

"Thanks, Max," Ben said. "It's good to be back. Please take us directly to Nob Hill . . ."

"How nice to be met with a limousine," Carolyn said. "That's something that would be easy to get used to . . ."

Ben laughed softly. "I totally agree."

During the flight the two had talked about Dr. Brunson and Allen, and the office. Still Carolyn somehow had the feeling that neither one of them was much on his mind. And it wasn't until after the small, intimate dinner served in the library that Ben began speaking what was truly on his mind.

"It still seems strange to me," he said, "that all of this is mine . . . Phineas Elias, Anne's grandfather, named Anne and myself as sole heirs. And at Anne's death it became mine . . ."

Carolyn noticed and was gratified that Ben no longer stumbled over the fact of Anne's death.

"Now I don't know what to do with it," Ben finished.

Not knowing what was coming next, Carolyn waited.

"It's not just the house and grounds," he said, "though they are extensive, as you can see. But, the whole estate . . ."

He reached across the table and took both her hands in his. "So, Carolyn, now that you've consented to share my life . . . I'd like you to help me to decide what to do with all this."

Despite herself, Carolyn's heart gave a lurch, but he wasn't finished yet.

"I don't want to sell it . . . and, at least for now, I'm not sure I want to live here . . ."

She was thoughtful. "Do you have *any* ideas about how best to utilize it?"

He answered slowly. "Yes, and I'd like your opinion . . ."

For the next few minutes Ben outlined his plan. His growing dream, he told Carolyn, had been to provide sort of a health retreat for individuals or husbands and wives, where they could get away from it all for a few days.

"Just to relax . . . recoup their energies . . ."

The Nob was large enough, and quiet enough, he explained, to handle a dozen or so such individuals or couples at the same time. "And the grounds are large enough for a number of people to have the privacy they need . . . to wander around, sit in the sun, read or swim. Or, whatever pleased them . . ."

He looked around him. "This library is a wonderful place to read. It's large and well lighted. I've already been moving some of Anne's books here . . . caring for one's own body. I'm getting a number of videos on the same subjects . . .

"All the meals served here will be . . . well, you know the way we eat. They'll be like that. And, if people want to learn, we'll teach them how to prepare food so they can live healthily."

Ben grinned boyishly. "I know I'm talking too much. But, I get very excited about the project. What do you think about all of this?"

"I think it's wonderful!" Carolyn said, clapping her hands. "This fine old home is a great for people to come to spend a few days. As you said, where they can, well . . . just rest and become rejuvenated . . ."

She hesitated, "But I do have just one tiny suggestion."

"What's that?"

"Well . . . the third floor suite . . ." Color rose to her cheeks. "Where we've talked of spending our honeymoon . . .?"

"Yes?"

"Let's keep it just the way it is. I'd like for us to come here as often as we can . . . so we can share in the healing of lives and bodies that I believe will take place here . . ."

Ben touched her fingertips to his lips. "Consider it done."

He arose from the table and took her hand. From the window they beheld an unfolding miracle. He pointed, "Watch the top of the Bridge . . ."

Carolyn looked. A solid bank of fog met her gaze. "Ben, I can't see the Bridge."

"Keep looking."

A wispy, gossamer fabric of mist unrolled and streamed past their eyes. Then another. Suddenly she saw it: the very topmost peak of the pylons, touched by a spot of gold. Layer after layer of fog was being stripped away, revealing the Bridge in all its glory — gilded by the setting sun.

"I see it, Ben. The Bridge, painted with gold. The *Golden Gate* Bridge! It's wonderful!"

"Yes," he said, "the gate is opening . . . to our future."

EPILOGUE

Washington, D. C. — The male secretary announced, "Mr. Rush, Senator Harold Ransom will see you now. Please follow me." He led Ben into the spacious office.

From behind the huge oak desk that dominated the otherwise Spartan room, a tall, distinguished-looking man arose and extended his hand. In that brief moment, Ben was struck by the curiously-wrought ring on the hand that gripped his: a death's head, with a scintillating diamond forming the skull.

"Mr. Rush, you have a rather notable ancestor in your family tree. Dr. Benjamin Rush holds a high place of honor in our nation's history . . ."

"Yes, sir, he does."

"Anyway — please be seated — I want to thank you for taking time to come to Washington . . ."

"Glad to be of service, Senator Ransom," Ben said, his eyes drawn again to the ring.

The Senator noted his gaze and smiled. "My ring . . .?" He touched it and then lightly traced the jagged scar on the left side of his face.

"Both of these — the scar and the ring — are souvenirs of Kenya. I served there a few years as ambassador," he explained. "And I happened to arrive in the country just in time for the Mau Mau uprising . . ."

He grinned wryly. "A case of being in the right place at the wrong time. The scar was the gift of a Mau Mau warrior who didn't appreciate my efforts to bring peace . . ."

"And the ring," he handed it to Ben for his inspection, "was a gift from Jomo Kenyatta, the country's first president. He gave it in appreciation for my efforts in his country's behalf."

Ben handed back the ring. "It's certainly striking."

"Yes. It never fails to attract attention." He picked up a note pad. "Well, let's get right to the matter at hand. May I call you Ben?"

"Of course."

"As you probably know, I have been elected chairman of the select committee, recently appointed by the Senate to investigate certain improprieties, having to do with the subject you cover so well in your forthcoming book . . ."

"I am surprised, Senator," Ben said, "my book isn't even off the press . . ."

"The Washington grapevine in this area is very active, Ben. And, frankly, some of the questions you have been asking of and about certain people and practices has come to our attention."

He laughed drily. "And, I might also add, your research has caused concern in the ranks of some of the, er, rather unethical persons who have cause to feel concern."

"I don't understand, Senator . . ."

The Senator's face assumed a serious demeanor. "To begin, let me say, this meeting is not in any way an interrogation. It's an informal chat. But, I'd like to know if you would be willing to appear before our select committee to answer some of the same questions I will be asking you? Except, at that time you might be requested to answer under oath . . ."

Ben hesitated briefly. "Yes, sir, I would be willing."

The Senator tapped the desk with his pencil before going on. "Ben, for your information, our committee has been investigating numerous methods of treating cancer, including alternatives. And, I was interested to note in this regard, that you make reference to a certain cancer industry, or cartel . . .?"

"Yes, sir, I did."

The Senator nodded thoughtfully. "I don't mind telling you that some of the questions you asked in your research are ones we should have been asking years ago . . ."

"Which questions, sir?"

"Questions dealing with the suppression of the truth as it relates to certain natural substances and healing arts . . ."

"I assume, Senator, that you are referring to such therapies as metabolic therapy, nutritional therapy, herbal therapy . . . ayurvedic therapies[65], hydrogen peroxide therapy, autouropathy[66], fasting therapy, homeopathy, naturopathy, electrotherapy[67], oxygen therapy[68] . . . and . . ."

The Senator chuckled, "You've certainly done your homework." "Yes, sir. It is true, I have been investigating the authenticity and validity of these and other therapies . . . all of which should *constitutionally*, be made available to the people as a matter of personal choice . . ."

"Hold it, Ben," the Senator said. "Don't run away with me. For the record, I am personally in agreement with you, as are many members of my committee . . ."

"Then what are we waiting for, Senator?" Ben asked, suddenly very angry, "People are dying out there . . . And because they don't have freedom of medical choice, the help that is available isn't adequate."

Dr. Anne's Journal

His voice choked. "My wife was among them . . ."

"Your wife was also a doctor," the Senator reminded.

"But she wasn't one of *them*!"

"What do you mean? Not one of them?"

"The ones that set themselves up as gods. Gods with the power to limit freedom of choice . . ."

His face became suffused with barely controlled anger. "Damn those would-be gods . . . the ones who prevent freedom of medical choice! Damn those delegates of the American Medical Association who refused to pass the patients' bill of rights . . . the very bill proposed by their own leadership!

"Damn them for their stand against answering their patients' questions! Questions dealing with basic information — costs, benefits . . . even the risks of treatments. For denying patients the right to obtain copies of their own health records, and 'protected communications' with doctors . . ."[69]

Ben drew a deep breath. "You asked me if I would be willing to testify before your committee. You bet your life I'm ready, and no pun intended. Just tell me where and when. I'll be there."

Clearly moved by Ben's tirade, the Senator didn't respond immediately. He shoved his chair back from his desk and began pacing back and forth across his office, his ring catching and reflecting the light from the late afternoon sun at every turn. How ironically fitting, Ben thought, that the man charged with this responsibility should be wearing such a ring . . .

When the Senator finally spoke, his voice was low with controlled emotion . . .

"Ben, I am terribly sorry about your wife. I understand how you feel . . . because I nearly lost my own private battle with cancer . . ."

For a full minute he appeared lost in thought.

Ben took a deep breath and let it out slowly. "Senator, you have personal knowledge of what I speak, don't you?"

The Senator blanched. "What do you mean?"

"You know what I mean," Ben said. "I am referring to a John Doe . . . who was treated at a certain cancer clinic. A man whose bill was paid in cash . . ."

Senator Ransom's grip on the chair arms tightened; his knuckles became the same color as his full head of white hair. The man's deep-set eyes, burned brightly with fury. "Ben Rush, don't ever utter those words outside this office!"

As quickly as the Senator's anger flashed, it was gone. Suddenly he leaped to his feet and stood in front of Ben. "We've got a tough job to do. A long, difficult investigation. And we need your help. That's why I asked you to come."

He cleared his throat and checked his notes. "First, let me tell you, your efforts haven't been entirely in vain. Largely as a result of your research, my committee is investigating Bertram Collins and his associations, business and otherwise, with Dr. Allen Drury . . .

"Furthermore," he went on, "we are investigating all the activities of BII, Bullion International, Inc., and Roger Keller, the chairman of the board of that institution, especially as it relates to the newly FDA-approved cancer drug, Oncoplex . . ."

He looked up, his face grim. "That's just the beginning. We're also investigating everything and everybody having to do with any and all of these persons and organizations and their possible interrelationships with each other . . ."

"That's all well and good, Senator," Ben said coldly, "but somehow it seems almost like an exercise in futility . . . too little, too late . . ."

"What do you mean?" the Senator demanded.

"You seem to be focusing on the mere tip of the iceberg, not the iceberg itself. BII and Collins are the tip. The cartels are the iceberg. And the controls wielded by the cartels under discussion are so vast as to defy description. At the moment I'm referring to the power they manifest through the media . . ."

Ben slapped the desk with the flat of his hand and continued vehemently, "Drugs, for instance. Few programs can be viewed on TV that aren't sponsored by over-the-counter drugs. Literally hundreds of hours each day are given over to the subtle messages that these OTC drugs are good for us. That they will fix almost anything . . .

"The average viewer has been so brainwashed by drugging messages that his or her response to illness is no longer rational. I call it the Pavlov's dog syndrome. Automatic reaction. 'If you're stressed out, reach for a pill.' 'If you've got a headache, reach for a pill.' The public hears that message so often they no longer think about it. They simply act. And swallow another handful of pills . . ."

In the intensity of his declaration, Ben began pacing. "It's no wonder our kids are on drugs. They're simply modeling their parents! A vicious cycle we've got to break!"

Suddenly embarrassed by his vehemence, Ben said, "Please forgive me, Senator, but my research into the causes and treatments of cancer has led me to believe that the causes of cancer are not simple. They are multiple. Excessive drugging is just one of them . . . and I am grateful that your committee is becoming concerned about that problem.

"But I have another concern that outweighs even that one. It's the problem *behind* the problems . . ."

"What's that?"

"It's money. The almighty dollar. It's the immense profits being made by the cancer-pharmaceutical industry. It's the *trillions* of dollars the industry is reaping from the life's blood of the millions of people dying of cancer . . ."

"That's a strong charge," the Senator warned.

"Strong, but true. Ask yourself why cancer research is so tightly controlled. It's to control the money. Ask yourself why new and inexpensive and public domain substances and modalities are denied legitimacy. It's to control the money!

"Why are thousands each year being forced to flee to other countries to receive treatment that's not permitted in the USA? Isn't money at the root of it all?"

Ransom suddenly stood, his knuckles upon his desk, leaning toward Ben. "Young man, has a little learning made you mad?" He jabbed a finger at Ben, the forceful gesture emphasized a thousand-fold by the scintillating diamond of his death's head ring. "Much of what you say is true. Perhaps most of it. But, there are two sides to every coin . . ."

Ben broke in with the challenge, "Such as?"

"You spoke of the trillions of dollars being raked in by the medical-pharmaceutical industry. And it may be true. But it's a trade off, Ben. A necessary trade off!"

"I don't understand . . ."

"I know you don't understand. That's why I'm asking you to carefully temper your remarks to the media. Much of that 'blood money,' as you inferred, is veritably the life blood for millions of families . . . because it provides them with jobs that put food on their tables and a shelter over their heads . . ."

A different picture flashed into Ben's mind: thousands of ordinary men and women caught in the web — with spouses and children to care for. Production workers in chemical labs and factories. Secretaries. Shipping clerks . . . and others. Most who would not have a job were it not for the vast army of patients dying of cancer . . .

Ben groaned, "How ironical!"

"True, Ben. It's ironical as hell, and just as necessary. Without being facetious, let me give you some facts."

He slammed one fist into the palm of the other. "If we were to find a cure for cancer today, and put it into effect tomorrow, within a few months our country would suffer the worst financial crisis of it's two-hundred year history!"

Ben gasped. "That can't be true!"

"Can't be, but it is. The war on cancer is like any other war. And just as hellish. Wars make money. Prosperity comes as a result of wars. Boom times always follow in the wake of wars. The war on cancer is no different . . ."

Their eyes locked for a long moment, neither man aware of the faint hum of traffic or the metronomic ticking of the clock.

Finally Ben broke the silence. "Are you telling me that there'll never be any hope for the victims of cancer?"

The Senator shook his head. "No, Ben, I'm not saying that."

"Are you saying, there's nothing at all we can do about this damnable situation?"

"No, I'm not saying that either . . ."

"Then what are you saying?"

"I'm saying there are things we can do that we're not presently doing. Or that we could do better. One, we can — all of us — begin taking full responsibility for our own health.

"Two, as a nation, we can change our focus from *curing* to *preventing*. Three, we can begin passing — and enforcing laws — that will outlaw massive pollution . . . pollution of all kinds. And, yes, we can pass laws that will give us freedom of medical choice."[70]

The Senator sat down slowly. "Ben, believe me, there is hope. Not for today. Perhaps not even tomorrow . . ." He spread his arms wide, ". . . but sometime in the future . . ."

His face softened. "Oh, and there is one more thing we can do . . .

"We can recreate the same driving force that brought our fathers to this new land . . . rekindle that same passionate desire to reject oppression of every kind . . ."

From where he sat, Ben's eyes converged upon the capitol dome, in the foreground a battlefield, strewn with the bitter results of battle: both overlaid by the careworn, skeletal face of Abraham Lincoln . . .

"The world . . . can never forget . . ." he was saying.

Have we forgotten? Ben wondered.

". . . a new nation, conceived in liberty and dedicated to the proposition that all men are created equal. . . . the nation shall, under God, have a new birth of freedom . . ."

New birth of freedom, Ben thought, *the freedom of health choices*. He turned. His eyes caught and held those of the Senator, a hopeful smile playing upon his lips. Ben nodded slightly . . .

MEDICAL DOCTORS SPEAK OUT

"Most of us at one time or another, have had to sit helplessly by and watch a loved one die of that dread disease, *cancer*. DR. ANNE'S JOURNAL will most assuredly awaken those feelings of despair and pain you have probably tried to forget. But those feelings may quickly turn to anger as you discover that your loved one may have suffered needlessly.

"The American public has been duped into believing that expensive surgery, radiation and chemotherapy are the only cancer treatments with any validity. Typical of one case mentioned in DR. ANNE'S JOURNAL, a patient can already be scheduled for surgery the next day, *before he has even been told that he has cancer*. Things are rushed so fast that the patient and his family have no time to gather their thoughts and consider all of the possibilities. If they should dare to ask about alternative treatments, such as laetrile, they are immediately intimidated and told not to even consider such absurdity. 'Such therapies are unproven,' they are told, when in fact, such therapies have been around in other countries for decades and have a very good track record.

"I have personally known many cancer victims who no longer have any trace of their disease, although at the time of their diagnosis, they were given only months or days to live. The key to the success of their treatments was the belief that all cancer is caused by metabolic imbalance of some kind and that the lumps, bumps and tumors are mere symptoms. Corrections of such imbalances allows the body to heal itself, as pointed out in DR. ANNE'S JOURNAL.

"What is it then that prevents us from even hearing of these remarkable results experienced by thousands? Isn't the whole world waiting with bated breath for a cure for cancer? Hardly. You may find this difficult to believe, but there are forces at work trying very hard not only to keep this information from the public, but also to stop enlightened doctors from helping their patients. DR. ANNE'S JOURNAL describes some of the antics and tactics used by special interest groups to sabotage the truth.

"Physicians who offer cancer patients alternative treatments and provide them with information on taking responsibility for their own health are often unjustly targeted by the local medical authorities. Offices have been raided and private patients' medical charts have been removed and scrutinized. Many doctors have had their medical license revoked and have been forced to relocate to continue their practice, some even out of the United States. These courageous doctors refused to compromise their medical principles by giving up what they knew would save their patients' lives. (This leads one to question what the so-called 'opposition' feels about those very same patients' lives, that they themselves couldn't help with 'proven' radiation, surgery or chemotherapy.)

"As outlined in DR. ANNE'S JOURNAL, one of the signers of the U.S. Declaration of Independence was an M.D., named Benjamin Rush. Dr. Rush would have been appalled at this blatant abuse of that segment of the Constitution intended to insure medical freedom and protect the patients' right to *life, liberty and the pursuit of happiness.*"

Sandra Denton, M.D., Omni Medical Center, 615 E. 82nd Avenue, Suite 300, Anchorage Alaska 99518. (907) 344-7775.

ANOTHER DOCTOR . . .

The publishers of ROGER'S RECOVERY FROM AIDS, a book I could not lay down until I had read the very last page, have done it again! I have heard these same words from many others to whom I have given or recommended they read ROGER'S RECOVERY. And now, they have produced DR. ANNE'S JOURNAL, another book that hooks the reader and demands his undivided attention for a spectacular, factual- and emotion-packed journey.

This book fills a big need. The need to teach people about the alternative methods available in the treatment of patients with degenerative diseases, especially cancer. In a subtle and balanced way, DR. ANNE'S JOURNAL weaves the intricate and emotional story of Dr. Anne, her family, friends and colleagues into a masterpiece of consciousness, awareness, understanding and knowledge!

Through love and understanding, this warm and caring book touches the heart and soul of the reader. With kindness and firmness the author presents through the characters of the story the powerful medical-pharmaceutical cartel and its firm grip on the disease-care system of the United States. I call this the marriage bond of the "Greed Disease," with the love of power and money being the root of evil.

Like its predecessor, ROGER'S RECOVERY . . ., DR. ANNE'S JOURNAL is a book that will be enjoyed by both lay people and professionals alike. It will serve to open the minds to both sides of medicine in the U.S. — conventional and alternative. With this realization, the individual may make a more intelligent choice in the type of medical care he wishes to receive or to practice.

Roy Kupsinel, M.D.
P.O. Box 550, Oviedo, FL 32765-0550
(407) 365-6681

ANOTHER DOCTOR . . .

Congratulations on DR. ANNE'S JOURNAL, a great book! It was hard to put down once I got into it. You surely have a way of getting right to the heart strings of your characters. Your portrayal of the mental anguish of cancer patients was very real.

Your insights into the behind-the-scenes politics, the skulduggery, the persecution and distresses of doctors who dare to think and be independent, who dare to follow total person restoration approaches and get rid of disease causes rather than just palliate, were just as real and accurate.

Reading DR. ANNE'S JOURNAL was to relive, even painfully, many of my own persecution experiences of 27 years ago. It was a salve to know that somebody really finally does understand and empathize.

I believe DR. ANNE'S JOURNAL will greatly help to open the eyes of a good many people. It will be a real and much needed encouragement for those searching for realistic understandings of how to choose and involve themselves with effective alternative therapies and how to live lifestyles that help control and eliminate their cancers.

I assure you that I will highly recomment DR. ANNE'S JOURNAL for any cancer patients I encounter in the future.

Leo Roy, M.D., N.D., F.A.N.A.
1075 Bernard Ave., Apt. 114
Kelowna, B.C. Canada V1Y 6P7
(604) 862-3228

NOTES

Chapter 5

1. Inlander, Charles B., Lowell S. Levin, Ed Weiner, *Medicine on Trial*, pp. 106, 113.

2. Cameron, Ewan and Linus Pauling, *Cancer and Vitamin C*, p. 206.

3. Salaman, Maureen. *Nutrition, The Cancer Answer*, p. 21.

4. Berger, Stuart, M.D. *What Your Doctor Didn't Learn in Medical School*, p. 32.

5. May 8, 1986.

Chapter Seven

6. See "The Drugging of America: our children," p. 39, *Health Freedom News*, June 1989.

7. Ibid, p. 2.

8. "Finally, After 11 Years, The Federal Court in Chicago, Illinois, Found The American Medical Association Guilty!!!" Motion Palpation Institute: Huntington Beach, California, 1987.

Chapter Nine

9. Mendelsohn, Robert S., M.D. *The Risks of Immunizations and How To Avoid Them*. The People's Doctor Newsletter, Inc.: Evanston, Illinois. 1988. Pages 3, 9, 38-39.

Chapter Eleven

10. Michael L. Culbert, D.Sc., is also the editor of *The Choice*, the official publication of the Committee for Freedom of Choice in Medicine, Inc., 1180 Walnut Avenue, Chula Vista, CA 92011.

Chapter Twelve

11. John M. Fink's *Third Opinion*, which is a comprehensive, "Interntional Directory to Alternative Therapy Centers for the Treatment and Prevention of Cancer. This book, along with other excellent materials concerning the treatment and prevention of cancer can be obtained by writing or calling, Cancer Control Society, 2043 N. Berendo St., Los Angeles, CA 90027. (213) 663-7801.

12. See Appendix II for a list of medical and freedom of medical choice lobbying groups with which you can also become involved to help make a difference.

Chapter 14

13. Richardson, John A., M.D., and Patricia Griffin, R.N. *Laetrile Case Histories, The Richardson Clinic Experience*. Bantam Books: New York. 1977. Pages 11-13.

14. Richardson, John, M.D., op cit., P. 10 ff.

15. Constitution of the United States, The Bill of Rights (Declared in force December 15, 1791), Article XIV.

Chapter Fifteen

16. *The Public Citizen Health Research Group Health Letter*, 2000 P St., NW, Washington, D.C., 20036.

17. National Health Federation, P.O. Box 688, Monrovia, CA 91016.

18. See Appendix II for further information on alternative healing therapy lobbying groups.

19. *The CHOICE, Official Publication of the Committee for Freedom of Choice in Medicine, Inc.*, 1180 Walnut Ave., Chula Vista, CA 92011.

Chapter Eighteen

20. Binger, Carl. *Revolutionary Doctor, Benjamin Rush.*

Chapter Nineteen

21. Published by W.B. Saunders Company, Harcourt Brace Jovanovich, Inc., Philadelphia. 1988.

22. Ibid, p. 104.

23. Richardson, John A., M.D. and Patricia Griffin. *Laetrile Case Histories, The Richardson Cancer Clinic Experience*. Bantam Books: New York. 1977.

24. Richardson and Griffin, op. cit.

25. Richardson & Griffin, op. cit.

26. Moss, Ralph W. *The Cancer Syndrome*. New York: Grove Press, 1980, p. 105.

Chapter Twenty

27. "In April 1970 the Food and Drug Administration assigned IND (Investigative New Drug) application number 6734 to the McNaughton Foundation, based in California, to test amygdalin-Laetrile. . . . Ten days later, permission was suddenly revoked by the FDA." Don C. Matchan, "A New Look at Laetrile," *Let's Live*, June 1973.

Chapter Twenty-One

28. Ordering information for all of these books is provided in Appendix I.

Chapter Twenty-Two

29. Moss, Ralph W. *The Cancer Syndrome*. Grove Press: New York, 1980, p. 16.

30. *The New England Journal of Medicine*, May 8, 1986. The full quote indicates that between the years of 1950 to 1982, "In the United States, these years were associated with increases in the number of deaths from cancer. . . . we are losing the war against cancer."

31. Mansell, Thomas H. *Cancer Simplified*. Woodlawn Press: Aliquippa, PA.

Chapter Twenty-Three

32. Mullins, Eustace. *Murder By Injection, The Story of The Medical Conspiracy Against America*. Staunton, Virginia: The National Council for Medical Research, 1988, p. 60.

33. Ibid, p. 62.

34. Moss, Ralph W., *The Cancer Syndrome*. Grove Press: New York. 1980, p. 133.

35. Moss, op. cit., pages 253-275.

36. U.S. Senate, July 1977 hearings on Health and Scientific Research.

37. Moss, ibid.

38. Griffin, G. Edward, *World Without Cancer*. American Media: Westlake Village, California. 1974. Page 501.

39. Moss, ibid.

40. This factual case history is detailed in *Laetrile Case Histories . . .*, by John A. Richardson, M.D., and Patricia Griffin, R.N., published by Bantam Books, New York, 1977.

Chapter Twenty-Four

41. California Business and Professional Code, Section 2146.

42. American Biologics-Mexico S.A., 1180 Walnut Avenue, Chula Vista, California 92011.

43. November 8, 1976.

44. Cameron, Ewan, M.B., Ch.B, F.R.C.S. (Glasgow), F.R.C.S. (Edinburgh) and Linus Pauling, Ph.D. *Cancer and Vitamin C, A Discussion of the Nature, Causes, Prevention, and Treatment of Cancer with Special Reference to the Value of Vitamin C.* The Linus Pauling Institute of Science and Medicine: Menlo Park, California, 1979.

45. Ibid., p. 80.

46. Ibid., p. 111.

47. Cameron and Pauling, op cit, p. 86.

48. Ibid., pp. 106-107.

49. Reference *Third Opinion, An International Directory to Alternative Therapy Centers for the Treatment and Prevention of Cancer*, John M. Fink; *Crackdown on Cancer*, Ruth Yale Long, Ph.D.; and *Alternative Cancer Therapies, Tijuana Clinics, Where and How To Go*, Sally Wolper.

50. Per telephone conversation with Michael L. Culbert, D.Sc., Chairman of the Board, Committee for Freedom of Choice in Medicine, Inc.

Chapter Twenty-Five

51. Fox, Arnold, M.D. and Barry Fox. *Immune For Life*. Prima Publishing and Communications: Rocklin, California, 1990. Page 26.

52. Ibid.

53. *Physicians' Desk Reference*. Medical Economics Company, Inc.: Oradell, N.J., 1989.

54. Griffin, H. Winter, M.D. *Complete Guide to Prescription & Non-Prescription Drugs*. The Body Press: Los Angeles, 1990.

55. Long, James W., M.D. *The Essential Guide To Prescription Drugs, 1980*. Harper & Row: New York, p. 698.

56. Long, Ruth Yale, Ph.D., op cit, p. 20 ff.

57. Sattilaro, Anthony J., M.D. *Recalled By Life, The Story of My Recovery From Cancer*. Houghton Mifflin Company: Boston, 1982.

58. Long, Ruth Yale, Ph.D., *Crackdown on Cancer*. Nutrition Education Association, Inc.: Houston, TX. 1983.

Chapter Thirty-Two

59. Chopra, Deepak, M.D. *Quantum Healing, Exploring the Frontiers of Mind/Body Medicine.* Bantam Books: New York, 1989. Page 19.

60. Siegel, Bernie S., M.D. *Love, Medicine and Miracles.* Harper & Row: New York, 1986.

61. Public lecture, Portland, Oregon, March 2, 1990.

Chapter Thirty-Three

62. *Alive and Well; Will Bible Foods Prevent Cancer?; Cooking for the Lord; and The Menu and The Mind,* all written by Mary June Parks and published by Parks Publishers, 315 Leawood Drive, Frankfort, Kentucky 40601.

63. Personal letter from Mary June Parks, dated February 19, 1990.

64. The names and address mentioned are listed in Appendix II.

Epilogue

65. Term describing ancient East Indian healing arts.

66. Margie Adelman, N.D., "Autouropathy," *Alternative Times* (January 1990).

67. U.S. House of Representatives, HR-12169, February 7, 1931.

68. "AIDS, Cancer, Cured by Hyperoxygenation," Waves Forest, *Health Freedom News*, June 1988.

69. "AMA Turns Down Patiens' Rights," *Health Letter*, February 1990. Report from the December 1989 Convention in Hawaii.

70. See Appendix II for list of freedom of choice in health therapies organizations.

APPENDIX I

Most books named in the body of the text and bibliography can be obtained from local libraries and well-stocked book stores, or both sources can obtain them for you. However, certain difficult-to-obtain books may be secured from the following suppliers:

- Cancer Control Society, 2043 N. Berendo Street, Los Angeles, CA 90027.

- Health Research, Mokelumne Hill, California 95245.

- BLI Publishing and Productions, 3960 Wilshire Blvd., Los Angeles, CA 90010-3306.

APPENDIX II

The following organizations are involved in the critical issue of securing our freedom of choice in healing therapies. By adding your voice, influence and financial means with them, you can become a vital part of the swelling grass roots movement dedicated to the purpose of gaining or regaining our Constitutional right to seek the healing therapy of our choice.

- American Natural Hygiene Society, P.O. Box 30630, Tampa, Florida 33630.

- Center for Science in the Public Interest, 1501 16th St., N.W., Washington, D.C. 20036-1499.

- Coalition for Alternatives in Nutrition and Healthcare, Inc. (CANAH), P.O. Box B-12, Richlandtown, PA 18955.

- National Health Federation, P.O. Box 688, Monrovia, CA 91016.

- Project CURE, 2020 K Street, NW, Suite 350, Washington, D.C. 20069.

- Public Citizen Health Research Group, 2000 P St., NW, Washington, D.C. 20036.

Appendix

- The Advancement of Alternate Choices in Healing
  Therapies (AACHT), 6939 Federal Blvd., No.
  311, Lemon Grove, CA 92045.

- The Committee for Freedom of Choice in Medicine,
  Inc., 1180 Walnut Ave., Chula Vista, CA
  92011.

SOURCES AND RESOURCES

Adelman, Margie, N.D. "Autouropathy," *Alternative Times* (January 1990).

Airola, Paavo O., Ph.D., N.D. *Cancer, Causes, Prevention and Treatment, The Total Approach.* Phoenix, Arizona: Health Plus, Publishers, 1963.

Allen, Hannah. *Don't Get Stuck, The Case Against Vaccinations and Injections.* Oldsmar, Florida: Natural Hygiene Press, 1985.

Anderson, Henry L.N., Ed.D., D.D., M.F.C.C. *Helping Hand, 8-Day Diet Programs for People Who Care About Wellness.* Inglewood, CA: Associated Family Counselors, 1986.

Antonio, Gene. *The AIDS Coverup?* San Francisco: Ignatius Press, 1986.

Barnhart, Edward, R., Publisher. *Physicians' Desk Reference, 43 Edition.* Oradell, N.J.: Medical Economics Company, Inc., 1989.

Bartnett, Beatrice, D.C., N.D. *Urine-Therapy.* Botsford, CT: Water of Life Publishing, 1989.

Bartnett, Beatrice, D.C., N.D. *The Miracles of Urine-Therapy.* Hollywood, FL: Water of Life, Publishing, 1987.

Dr. Anne's Journal

Benson, Herbert, M.D., with William Proctor. *Beyond the Relaxation Response*. New York: Berkley Books, 1986.

Benson, Herbert, M.D., with Mariam Z. Klipper. *The Relaxation Response*. New York: Avon Books, 1976.

Berger, Stuart, M.D. *What Your Doctor Didn't Learn in Medical School*. New York: William Morrow and Company, 1988.

Berkow, Robert, M.D., Editor-in-Chief and Andrew J. Fletcher, M.B., B.Chir., Assistant Editor. *The Merck Manual, Fifteenth Edition*. Rahway, N.J.: Merck, Sharp & Dohme Research Laboratories, 1987.

Binger, Carl. *Revolutionary Doctor, Benjamin Rush*. New York: W.W. Norton Co., Inc., 1966.

Borell, George. *The Peroxide Story*. Anaheim, CA: George Borell Publisher, 1986.

Bradford, Robert W., D.Sc., Henry W. Allen and Michael L. Culbert, D.Sc. *The Biochemical Basis of Live Cell Therapy*. Chula Vista, CA: The Robert W. Bradford Foundation, A Trust, 1986.

Bradford, Robert W., D.Sc., Henry W. Allen and Michael L. Culbert, D.Sc. *Oxidology, The Study of Reactive Oxygen Toxic Species (ROTS) and Their Metabolism in Health and Disease*. Los Altos, CA: The Robert W. Bradford Foundation, A Trust, 1985.

Bruce, Gene. "The Drugging of America: our children," *Health Freedom News, The Journal of the National Health Federation*, June 1989.

_____, *California Business and Professional Code*, Section 2146.

Buttram, Harold E., M.D. *Vaccinations and Immune Malfunction*. Quakertown, PA: The Humanitarian Publishing Company, 1985.

Cameron, Ewan, M.B., Ch.B., F.R.C.S. (Edinburgh and Glasgow), and Linus Pauling, Ph.D. *Cancer and Vitamin C*. Menlo Park, California: Linus Pauling Institute of Science and Medicine, 1979.

_____, *The CHOICE*, Official Publication of the Committee for Freedom of Choice in Medicine, Inc., 1180 Walnut Ave., Chula Vista, CA 92011.

Chopra, Deepak, M.D. *Quantum Healing, Exploring the Frontiers of Mind/Body Medicine*. New York: Bantam Books, 1989.

_____, "Constitution of the United States, The Bill of Rights, Article XIV."

Culbert, Michael L., D.Sc. *Freedom From Cancer*. Seal Beach, California: '76 Press, 1974.

Culbert, Michael L., D.Sc. *Save Your Life*. Virginia Beach/Norfolk, Virginia: The Donning Company, Publishers, 1983.

Diamond, Harvey and Marilyn. *Fit for Life*. New York: Warner Books, 1985.

Diamond, Harvey and Marilyn. *Living Health*. New York: Warner Books, 1987.

_____, "Finally, After 11 Years, The Federal Court in Chicago, Illinois, Found the American Medical Association Guilty!!!" Motion Palpation Institute: Huntington Beach, California, 1987.

Elben. *Vaccination Condemned*. Los Angeles: Better Life Research, 1981.

Fink, John M. *Third Opinion, An International Directory to Alternative Therapy Centers for the Treatment and Prevention of Cancer*. Garden City Park, New York: Avery Publishing Group, Inc., 1988.

Forest, Waves, "AIDS, Cancer Cured by Hyperoxygenation," *Health Freedom News*, June 1988.

Fox, Arnold, M.D. and Barry Fox. *Immune for Life*. Rocklin, CA: Prima Publishing and Communications, 1990.

Giller, Robert M., M.D. and Kathy Matthews. *Medical Makeover*. New York: Warner Books, 1986.

Govani, Laura E., Ph.D., R.N. and Janice E. Hayes, Ph.D., R.N. *Drugs and Nursing Implications, Edition 4*. Norwalk, Connecticut: Appleton-Century-Crofts, 1982.

Gregory, Scott, O.M.D. and Bianca Leonardo, N.M.D. *They Conquered AIDS, True Life Adventures*. Palm Springs, CA: Tree of Life Publications, 1989.

Griffin, G. Edward. *World Without Cancer, The Story of Vitamin B-17*. Westlake Village, California: American Media, 1974.

Griffin, H. Winter, M.D. *Complete Guide to Prescription & Non-Prescription Drugs*. Los Angeles: The Body Press, 1990.

Hausman, Patricia & Judith Benn Hurley. *The Healing Foods, The Ultimate Authority on the Curative Power of Nutrition.* Emmaus, PA: Rodale Press, 1989.

Hovnanian, Ralph R., B.S., M.S. *Cancer Alternative Therapies' Cure Rates.* Huntington, Connecticut: Natural Hygiene, Inc., 1985.

Hutchinson, Michael. *The Book of Floating, Exploring the Private Sea.* New York: William Morrow and Company, 1984.

Illich, Ivan. *Medical Nemesis, The Expropriation of Health.* New York: Pantheon Books, 1976.

Inlander, Charles B., Lowell S. Levin, Ed.D., and Ed Weiner. *Medicine on Trial.* New York: Prentice Hall Press, 1988.

Jones, Rochelle. *The Supermeds, How the Big Business of Medicine Is Endangering Our Health Care.* New York: Charles Scribner's Sons, 1988.

Kalokerinos, Archie, M.D. *Every Second Child.* New Canaan, Connecticut: Keats Publishing, Inc. 1974.

Long, Ruth Yale, Ph.D. *Crackdown on Cancer with Good Nutrition.* Houston, Texas: Nutrition Education Association, Inc., 1983.

Long, James W., M.D. *The Essential Guide To Prescription Drugs.* New York: Harper & Row, 1980.

Lynes, Barry, with John Crane. *The Cancer Cure That Worked! Fifty Years of Suppression.* Toronto, Canada: Marcus Books, 1987.

McDougall, John A., M.D. and Mary A. McDougall. *The McDougall Plan.* Piscataway, N.J.: New Century Publishers, 1983.

Manner, Harold W., Ph.D. *Facts About Metabolic Therapy.* San Ysidro, CA: Metabolic Research Foundation.

Mansell, Thomas H. *Cancer Simplified.* Aliquippa, Pennsylvania: Woodlawn Press, 1977.

Matchan, Don C. "A New Look at Laetrile," *Let's Live,* June 1973.

McDougall, John A., M.D. *McDougall's Medicine, A Challenging Second Opinion.* Piscataway, N.J.: New Century Publishers, 1985.

Mendelsohn, Robert S. M.D. *Male Practice, How Doctors Manipulate Women.* Chicago: Contemporary Books, Inc., 1982.

Mendelsohn, Robert S., M.D. *The Risks of Immunizations and How To Avoid Them.* The People's Doctor Newsletter, Inc.: Evanston, Illinois, 1988.

Mendelsohn, Robert S., M.D., George Crile, M.D., Samuel Epstein, M.D., Henry Heimlich, M.D., Alan Scott Levin, M.D., Edward R. Pinckney, M.D., David Spodick, M.D., Richard Moskowitz, M.D. and Gregory White, M.D. *Dissent In Medicine, Nine Doctors Speak Out.* Chicago: Contemporary Books, Inc., 1985.

Morgan, Brian L.G., Dr. *Nutrition Prescription.* New York: Fawcett Crest, 1987.

Morra, Marion & Eve Potts. *Choices, Realistic Alteratives in Cancer Treatment*. New York: Avon Books, 1987.

Moss, Ralph W. *The Cancer Syndrome*. New York: Grove Press, Inc., 1980.

Mullins, Eustace. *Murder by Injection, The Story of the Medical Conspiracy Against America*. Staunton, Virginia: The National Council for Medical Research, 1988.

Nelkin, Dorothy and Laurence Tancredi. *Dangerous Diagnostics, The Social Power of Biological Information*. New York: Basic Books, Inc., Publishers, 1989.

Newbold, H.L., M.D. *Vitamin C Against Cancer*. New York: Stein and Day, 1981.

Olsen, Kristin Gottschalk. *The Encyclopedia of Alternative Health Care*. New York: Pocket Books, 1989.

_____, *National Health Federation*, P.O. Box 688, Monrovia, CA 91016.

Oswald, Jean A., and Herbert M. Shelton, Ph.D. *Fasting for the Health of It*. Pueblo, Colorado: Nationwide Press, Ltd., 1983.

Parks, Mary June. *The Menu and the Mind*. Frankfort, Kentucky: Parks Publishers, 1986.

Paul, Michele, R.N. *The Women's Pharmacy*. New York: Simon & Schuster, 1983.

Potts, Eve and Marion Morra. *Understanding Your Immune System*. New York: Avon Books, 1986.

_____, *The Public Citizen Health Research Group Health Letter*, 2000 P St., NW, Washington, D.C. 20036.

Richardson, John A., M.D., and Patricia Griffin, R.N. *Laetrile Case Histories, The Richardson Cancer Clinic Experience*. Toronto/New York/London: Bantam Books, 1977.

Salaman, Maureen. *Foods That Heal*. Menlo Park, California: Statford Press, 1989.

Sattilaro, Anthony J., M.D. *Recalled By Life, The Story of My Recovery From Cancer*. Boston: Houghton Mifflin Company, 1982.

Shelton, Herbert M., Ph.D. *Fasting Can Save Your Life*. Bridgport, CN: Natural Hygiene Press, 1978.

Siegel, Bernie S., M.D. *Love, Medicine and Miracles*. New York: Harper & Row, 1986.

Siegel, Bernie S., M.D. *Peace, Love and Healing*. New York: Harper & Row, 1989.

Silverman, Milton, Ph.D., Phillip R. Lee, M.D., and Mia Lydecker. *Prescriptions for Death, The Drugging of the Third World*. Berkeley and Los Angeles, California: University of Los Angeles Press, 1982.

Thakkar, G.K. *Wonders of Uropathy*. Bombay, India: United Arts B.G. Kher Marg, 1989.

Tilden, John H., M.D. *Toxemia, The Basic Cause of Disease*. Bridgport, Connecticut: Natural Hygiene Press, 1982.

Urdang, Laurence, Editor in Chief, and Helen Harding Swallow, Managing Editor. *Mosby's*

Medical & Nursing Dictionary. St. Louis,
Missouri: The C.V. Mosby Co., 1983.

_____, U.S. House of Representatives, HR-12169,
February 7, 1931.

_____, "Hearings on Health and Scientific
Research," U.S. Senate, July 1977.

Wagman, Richard J., M.D., F.A.C.P., Editor. *The New
Complete Medical and Health Encyclopedia*.
Chicago: J.G. Ferguson Publishing Co., 1989.

Walford, Roy L., M.D. *The 120-Year Diet*. New York:
Simon & Schuster, 1986.

Wohl, Stanley, M.D. *The Medical Industrial Complex*.
New York: Harmony Books, 1984.

Wolper, Sally. *Alternative Cancer Therapies, Tijuana
Clinics, Where and How To Go*. La Mirada,
California: La Mirada Publications, 1983.

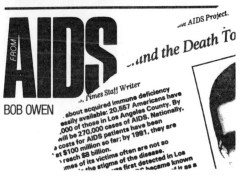